CHANGING THE CULTURE
for
DEMENTIA CARE

*The Path to a Better Quality of Life
for People with Alzheimer's Disease*

By Randy L. Griffin, RN, MS, HNC

PHC
PUBLISHING
GROUP

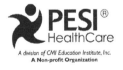

PESI®
HealthCare
A division of CMI Education Institute, Inc.
A Non-profit Organization

EAU CLAIRE, WISCONSIN
2012

For information on this and other
PESI HealthCare products
please call 800-843-7763 or
visit our website at www.pesihealthcare.com

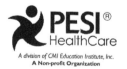

Cover: Shannon Gale
Back Cover Image: Tim Griffin
Editor: Barb Caffrey

"This wonderful book serves as a manual and a text for the student and the trainer from which quality interpersonal skills can be learned and blended with necessary care-giving approaches. There is much power in the inherent philosophy presented in this book. We all deserve to be treated with respect and dignity and with a deep understanding of our unique Selves. When this happens, a whole new caring world rewards us all."

Harry E. Morgan, MD
President
The Center for Geriatric and Family Psychiatry, Inc.
Glastonbury, Connecticut

"Randy's wisdom and insight into the challenges and leadership needed for culture change in dementia care are right on target. She uses patients' stories and scenarios to illuminate what we need to be mindful of in our daily caregiving... This book is a gem."

Cathy Nager MA, MPH
Elder Horizons Coordinator
Yale-New Haven Hospital

"All of the wonderful concepts are here to help individuals with dementia. Now, more people can become better caregivers, be present in their world, and enjoy their time together."

Betsy Clark, RN, BSN
Vice President and Clinical Supervisor
Regional Hospice and Home Care of Western Connecticut

Dedication

I would like to dedicate this book:

To the individuals and their families whose lives have been so greatly impacted by dementia. They became my teachers, and I became their most grateful student, learning firsthand about the true meaning of love, patience and courage. Most importantly, they taught me about the true meaning of life and why each day on this earth is so precious. Several of these individuals—Roger, Dick, Eddie and Carol—will stay close to my heart forever, for my work has been forever enriched by their presence in my life.

To my colleagues who continue to make important inroads in dementia care. Betsy Clark, Barbara Dondero, Carolyn De Rocco, Jeanne Kessler, Nancy Leonard, Irene Oday, Cathy Nager and Ana Nelson dedicate their daily lives to this cause. Dr. Harry Morgan has enlightened me about the journey dementia can take us on, all with a kind and caring presence.

To the many healthcare professionals who have influenced my work. From my first mentor 20 years ago whose leadership and vision continue to inspire me today, to the administrators, nurses and caregiving staff and all the team members who continually welcome me into their facilities, together we're finding new ways to improve care for people who have dementia.

To my good friends who offer their constant and unwavering support: Barbara Steinau, Alice Raim, Vicky Crompton and Richard Griffin provided me with loving critiques and thoughtful editing suggestions as I wrote this book. Lina Chase, Carol Jacoby, Gwen Wayne listened with open hearts as only friends can. My writing coach, Kevin Sylvester, helped to guide me with patience, kindness and a deep understanding of the importance of this book.

To my caring, supportive family who believed in me—and my work—from the very beginning.

And lastly, to my husband, Tim, who has dedicated his life's work to help change the culture for people with disabilities. I am truly fortunate to have such a compassionate, understanding partner on this journey who shares my belief that everyone deserves a quality of life worth living.

Foreword

Alzheimer's disease and dementing illnesses are the epidemic of the 21st century. If you are reading this book, you already know that. The hope of research is to find a cure. The reality is that these are complex syndromes of a failing brain. More than two dozen genes have been identified as possibly contributing to these diseases. We still do not understand the actual cause of this illness. This does not suggest there will be one cure found, and if so certainly not soon. At best we now have only palliative medication treatment available. Even if a magical cure to stop the development of Alzheimer's disease were found today, we still have millions of people living with the disease. Students often then conclude that these diseases are not treatable. Nothing could be further from the truth. We can intervene in many ways in people's lives—without curing, but still with great benefit. To do this, we must start with an understanding of the people with the illness.

People with Alzheimer's disease and other dementias are just that—people. They have personal histories alive within themselves. Their Selves survive even as they lose their skills for daily life. Each person has a unique blend of personhood and neurobiology waiting to be understood. Recent research suggests that the tone of communicating with a patient can dramatically change the emotional response of the patient, even in persons with advanced dementia where expressive verbal skills are meager. Patients spoken to in condescending tones (elderspeak) or patients who are treated as inanimate objects are more likely to react with anger, depletion and "resistance" to care. The personal experience of daily living is at the core of our sense of personal competence, autonomy and pleasure. When we are dependent upon others for this type of care, we also become dependent upon the "care-giving other" for these basic emotional needs. But, providing person-centered care is often challenging for us as care providers. The demands of our jobs, the sense of time pressures placed upon all in healthcare—and even our personal life situations—all create challenges to our ability to sensitively and empathically engage with our patients in their world and their internal space. Teaching care providers to engage and participate effectively in simple daily tasks with patients with dementia is often thought of as basic and even trivial. It is not!

Randy Griffin has undertaken this book to educate and train those who provide such vital and delicate care to people with dementia. With great wisdom from her years of personal professional caring and training of caregivers, she has created this work. Dignity, respect and sharing are emphasized. By using our own inner sense of Self, we become more authentic in meeting both the needs of our patients and also in growing our Selves. Viewing this partnership of patient and caregiver is truly a culture change in dementia care. The author weaves case vignettes throughout her book to illustrate the needs of people and the outcomes of the changing approaches to care and communication. Her approach looks beyond verbal interactions, carefully examining non-verbal moments of interpersonal exchange. The behaviors of patients, which are often challenging for caregivers, are then seen with a new focus that helps us understand the behavior and offers insight for changing these behaviors. Sources of distress are traced to their inner experiences such as pain, inner feeling tones or somatic sensations.

Team interactions provide support for the caregiver and offer insights for creative solutions in challenging situations. Working together can help make care settings become more like a comfortable and safe "home." This can soothe distressed patients who are frightened at their own loss of inner boundaries. The simple "feeling of family" can be enhanced with changes to the physical environment. An adaptive world for the cognitively impaired person is the goal. The centerpiece of this family life is often the dining table. Randy clearly and effectively offers a full menu of approaches to improving this social dining experience for the persons involved—patients and staff alike. And, this tightened sense of togetherness and security is reflected in the quality of life experience for all.

As a Medical Director of a premier Dementia Care nursing center, a consultant to outstanding Assisted Living residential care and a Geriatric Psychiatrist for people with dementia in their homes, I have personally seen the critical need for quality training of nursing assistants, personal care attendants, nurses and even physicians. Too painfully, I have also seen the plight of patients who are not fortunate enough to be cared for in programs with such skilled humane care. No expert medical or psychiatric consultant can cure or even treat the distress wrought by mediocre care providers. This wonderful book serves as a manual and a text for the student and the trainer from which quality interpersonal skills can be learned and blended with necessary caregiving approaches. There is much power in the inherent philosophy presented in this book. We all deserve to be treated with respect, dignity and with a deep understanding of our unique Selves. When this happens, a whole new caring world rewards us all.

Great work, Randy!

Harry E. Morgan, MD President,
The Center for Geriatric and Family Psychiatry, Inc.
Glastonbury, Connecticut
June, 2011

Table of Contents

Introduction

Buddha once said, *"You cannot travel the path
until you have become the path itself."*

I thought about what Buddha said when I sat down to write this book. It's similar to the saying "walk a mile in my shoes" in that you should try to understand someone before you criticize them. For centuries, we've been told that you need to experience a facet of life to truly know what it's like to live that experience. When we talk about dementia, however, odds are that none of you reading this book have experienced this condition, yet you're responsible for providing care for people who have dementia as it's become their way of life.

For most of us, "quality of life" has become something we take for granted. We go about our regular workday routines and family lives from day to day without giving much of what we do a second thought. Of course, much of what we do has been made easier by technological advances. We sit down at our Mac or PC to get the latest news without having to wait for the newspaper to be delivered. We can even send an email from our cell phone when we're far away from our computer. We've come to accept that things change every second of every day.

While technology continues to change the way we live, it's also brought major changes to the healthcare arena. For example, diagnostic imaging has become more accurate. Robots have been used to assist with surgery in treating prostate cancer, and some intelligent prosthetics can reputedly even "think." It's widely known that these advancements in medical care have greatly increased people's lifespans.

Yet as people live longer, they are more at risk for developing dementia. Today, one out of every two people over the age of 85 will be diagnosed with some form of dementia. Alzheimer's disease is the leading cause of dementia, the sixth-leading cause of death in the United States—and the only cause of death that cannot be prevented, cured or even slowed. From 2000–2006, for example, Alzheimer's disease deaths increased 46.1 percent, while other causes of death, such as stroke, HIV and heart disease, actually decreased.(1)

With a rapidly aging "Baby Boomer" population, Alzheimer's disease undoubtedly will continue to impact more lives. The nation's first "Baby Boomer" only became eligible for Social Security benefits in January 2008. Totaling more than 80 million, the "boomers" are the largest and wealthiest generation in U.S. history. When you combine the growing number of senior "boomers" with the increased number of reported deaths related to Alzheimer's disease, it's clear that new approaches to providing dementia care are sorely needed.

We're starting to know more about the onset of dementia and Alzheimer's disease. New studies are testing drugs that may, in our lifetimes, slow the onset of the disease. This news is hopeful, with implications that could be astounding. Still, I wonder why similar attention hasn't been paid to the manner in which we provide care for the 5 million people affected by Alzheimer's disease and related dementias today.

Innovation: What Innovation?

As a healthcare professional who has worked with people who have dementia and Alzheimer's disease for more than 30 years, I am frustrated by the lack of innovation and progress in the field of dementia. Little has changed over the years in terms of training, education and overall care; little has been done to actually "walk a mile" in the shoes of an individual with dementia.

If anything, dementia care has evolved in a backward fashion: individuals with cognitive impairments were brought into institutional settings with pre-established processes and systems. The care was not tailored toward the treatment of dementia as much as the individuals with dementia were forced to "fit in" with the system.

Remember that quote from Buddha: "You cannot travel the path until you have become the path itself."

What's the root of this problem? If we don't have a clear-cut path to lead us to a better way of providing care, then we can't help coming up against roadblocks. And roadblocks are exactly what we face today.

Institutional barriers prevent us from advancing the quality of care in this area. Think about the lack of mandatory training for healthcare workers in the field of dementia care. American medical schools don't require training in geriatric care, even though they are required to have clinical experience in obstetrics and pediatrics. Does this lack of a training mandate reflect a deeper prevailing view that individuals with dementia have little value to society as human beings? Is it based on the ill-conceived notion that if someone isn't complaining, then the process doesn't need to be changed? Or does anyone believe that the staff wouldn't benefit from ongoing, specialized training?

The reason I wrote this book is simple: individuals with dementia deserve better. And we, as healthcare providers, need to cut a swath through the system of inadequate care that exists today and establish a viable path toward care that focuses on the person—not simply the disease.

This philosophy is similar to that of the hospice movement introduced in the 1960s by British physician Dame Cicely Saunders and Dr. Elisabeth Kubler-Ross. They brought the subject of dying into the open, contending that individuals with terminal cancer needed to be treated as unique human beings with individual needs and rights who deserved respect. The Connecticut Hospice, the first of its kind to open in the U.S., was the forerunner of the hospice care model that spread throughout the country. My dream is to see a similar focus on individuals with dementia so that "intentional caregiving" becomes the standard for care in this area.

As you've probably realized, this book is not intended to be a "Dementia 101" primer. There are plenty of books available that cover the basics of caring for people with dementia. This book takes that philosophy of "caring" one step further.

You'll see an ongoing theme throughout these pages: everything we do as caregivers needs to be performed intentionally, with care. Whether it's assisting a person with a daily task like bathing, eating, or applying lotion with the touch of our hands, we need to purposefully remember to be gentle, to be soothing, and to be kind in the way we provide care.

I believe firmly that specialized training is needed for all individuals who care for people with dementia. This training should recognize the value of every human being, and recognize that every individual, whether or not the person has dementia, possesses needs similar to our own. They need to feel loved, secure, respected and fulfilled. Above all, our patients need to feel a sense of belonging along with a sense of self worth.

How Do We Change the Current Mindset?

When I think about "walking a mile in the shoes" of someone with dementia, my feet start to ache. Here's why: for years, we've ignored the specific needs of those with cognitive impairments in favor of doing things the way we've always done. (I've seen this more often than I care to say.) But how does that help a person who has dementia? It's like stuffing a size 9 foot into a size 7 shoe because we like the way the shoe looks, even if it doesn't fit. The end result is a foot that's trying in vain to conform—swollen, with blisters, and on the brink of infection.

This outmoded mindset also establishes unfair expectations of our care staff. How can they possibly understand how to best provide care for people who have dementia without a system that requires advanced mandatory training focused on dementia caregiving? Roughly half of the fifty states do not require any type of formalized training for workers in dementia units. Of the remaining states, some require as few as two hours each year.(3) I find this incredible, given the fact that manicurists are required to have 400 hours of training before they are certified. Why haven't we demanded that same standard for our staff, who work with individuals with dementia?

In this book, I will use examples from my work to show how dementia care units can provide this level of care through a framework that meets each individual's needs in a specialized, humane way. I'll draw on the experiences I've had in my 30 year career—one that spans nursing, food service, healthcare administration and program development—to validate my assertions.

In my consulting practice today, my approach centers on treating the whole person, not just his or her symptoms, by creating a culture rich with emotional nourishment. (This is my book's approach as well.) Why? Because as caregivers, we're taught to do many tasks, but the manner in which we carry out those tasks is vital to our caregiving.

Individuals with dementia may have lost the ability to understand words, to verbalize their needs, or to express themselves. Everything in their world becomes disconnected, and it's our role to find ways to re-connect them to the world around them. This requires not only heightened awareness, but also true "intentional" caregiving on the part of the caregiver.

The path we're about to embark on is not an easy walk in the park. It requires us to make a commitment to see it through in order to make a true cultural change. By picking up this book, you've taken the first step on a journey toward creating a sustained change—a change in dementia care that is long overdue.

Chapter 1

History of Dementia and Methods of Care

Though there is no clear-cut path to optimal care models for individuals with dementia, a supportive culture needs to form the foundation before true construction can begin. The word "culture" may seem to be an odd one, but it's used in the same sense as T.S. Eliot used it here: "Culture may be described simply as that which makes life worth living."(4) When we think about this definition in the context of dementia care, it drives home a simple point: if we can't make a person's life worth living, then what are we doing?

Before we can even start to think about transforming the culture for dementia care, we need to understand two basic concepts: the definition of dementia and the past methods of treatment for individuals with this disease.

In terms of a definition, dementia can best be described as a loss of cognitive function—known as cognition—due to changes in the brain caused by disease or trauma. The changes may occur gradually or quickly; how they occur may determine whether the type of dementia is treatable or not. When we refer to cognition, we're referring to the act or process of thinking, perceiving and learning. Cognitive functions are often affected by dementia and may include one or more of the following:

- Decision making / judgment
- Memory
- Spatial orientation
- Thinking / reasoning
- Verbal communication

Alzheimer's disease, a form of dementia, is a progressive, chronic brain disorder that gradually destroys an individual's ability to learn, reason, make judgments, communicate and carry out daily activities. More than 5.3 million Americans suffer from Alzheimer's disease today, and estimates show that number could increase to between 11 and 16 million by 2050.(5) Even worse, an individual with the disease can live three to 20 years from the time the symptoms first appear. As the "Baby Boom" generation begins to turn 60, estimates show that someone in America develops Alzheimer's disease every 70 seconds—yes, every 70 seconds!

Using the definition of dementia I just described, think about T.S. Eliot's description of culture again. Do you see how the two are connected? If we want to truly make life worth living for people with dementia, then dementia care models need to evolve far more quickly than they have over the past 40 years. Considering the fact that we know so much more than we did even 10 years ago—and the fact that people are living longer lives—we are obligated to begin this transformation.

Dementia Care in the Past and Present

It would be an overstatement to say that treatment models in the past focused on quality of life. In fact, I'd go as far as to say that in some cases, treatment methods of the not-too-distant past were not even humane.

Years ago, we would take care of people with dementia by placing them in psychiatric institutions. During the 1970s, a custodial model emerged. Basically it went something like this: we took care of the patients' physical bodies, we fed and clothed them, and we gave them shelter —but we used physical and chemical restraints to make people comply with the treatment.

From those modest beginnings, the model evolved into more of a patient/doctor model in the 1980s. We still used physical restraints, but we did this out of a need to protect the patient. We didn't want patients to walk around disoriented, for fear that they might fall and hurt themselves. We felt that by using "reality orientation," the patients would eventually "get it." That is, if we told them over and over again what day it was, we could eventually bring them back to the "here and now." But did it work? Of course not!

In the 1990s, we began to see the emergence of a more socially aware model. It was then that the language of our profession started to change. We began calling patients "residents" and started offering myriad recreational activities to get rid of "empty hands"—residents sitting there all day with nothing to do. Slowly, we started to see more programs evolve, such as therapies involving pets, music, aromas and art. As the programs developed, however, their effective implementation proved to be difficult. It was unrealistic to think that a recreation director overseeing 30 or more residents at one time could keep everyone engaged. It furthered the belief that the nursing staff cared for the residents physical needs while the recreation staff took care of keeping everyone involved and happy.

A Breakthrough: Validation Therapy

It was during the 1990s that a breakthrough in dementia treatment came in the form of "Validation Therapy," founded by Naomi Feil. Born in Munich in 1932, Feil grew up in the Montefiore Home for the Aged in Cleveland, Ohio, where her father was the administrator and her mother was the head of the Social Service Department. After getting her MSW degree, she began working with the elderly and developed Validation Therapy in response to her dissatisfaction with the traditional methods of working with the elderly suffering from dementia. As recently as fifteen years ago, professionals in the field of dementia care were familiar with her work.

What is Validation Therapy? Basically, it's just as it sounds: it validates the thoughts, feelings and expressions of individuals with dementia. With this therapy, we caregivers can join with them in their "reality"—that is, whatever time they think they are at in their lives. This is a practice that should be a core component of every dementia care unit; unfortunately, I've found during the course of my work that many attendees at training sessions I lead aren't familiar with this therapy at all. I find that disturbing, as

Feil's work remains ground-breaking to this day. For more information about Validation Therapy, I encourage you to visit their website (*See Additional Resources*, **Websites**).

Today we find ourselves in the 21st Century with models bearing the descriptors "person-centered care," "relationship-centered care," and "integrated care." These models are more informed than past models and begin to get at the heart of why things need to change.

We now know that people with dementia or Alzheimer's disease begin to experience structural changes in the brain years before any signs of memory loss.[6] It's been medically proven that an individual's brain and nerve cells change during Alzheimer's disease. Over time, the brain shrinks dramatically, affecting nearly all of its functions. Nerve cell connections are lost, causing physical damage to certain pathways in the brain. These pathways are essential for thinking, learning and memorizing. Research has shown that the one part of the brain that stays intact throughout the disease is called the amygdala—it's the part of the brain that feels emotions, elicits emotions and perceives emotions. The amygdala, therefore, is what enables us to connect to the individual: it's the direct link to the person who exists within this illness until the very end of his or her life. With this clear proof in hand that we can continue to reach people with dementia, it's our responsibility to find a way to connect to the human being inside.

A Breakdown in Communications

Dementia impairs a person's ability to communicate effectively. Let's think about this a bit more. According to the Alzheimer's Association, the disease reduces a person's ability to decode and understand information, as well as decreases the ability to commit things to memory and express information. A person's ability to reconcile his or her external actions through internal speech is also reduced, effectively reducing the person's capacity to plan, problem-solve and reason.[7]

It's important to understand that the disease affects different parts of the brain at different times. As caregivers, we should constantly be looking to determine what abilities an individual exhibits and try to build upon them. Often we look at what a person can't do instead of what he or she still can do. If you're a caregiver, I'd like you to give serious thought to the following questions and try to answer them for the residents under your care.

- How has the disease affected the person's vision? For example, can they see what's on TV?
- Is the person able to track movement with their eyes? Sometimes the disease causes damage to the peripheral vision.
- Does the person have macular degeneration? Cataracts? Do they need glasses for distance or reading? Is their prescription for glasses up to date?
- Can the person hear well? Do they need a hearing aid? Have they used one in the past?
- Can the person see and recognize pictures?
- Can the person read? Do they understand simple instructions?
- Does the person mimic behavior?

Shouldn't having this knowledge about the individual influence the approach we take, the activities we design and the interactions we have with this person in general? A while back, I was working with a group of non-verbal residents with dementia at a long-term care facility. One day at lunch, I happened to be wearing a name tag. This prompted one of the gentlemen at the table to look at me and say, "Randy!" He was able to read my name tag, process the information and verbalize it. Truly amazing! No one thought he could read—never mind speak! That was the first clue we had that he could still read. Sadly, sometimes we simply assume that people with dementia have no skills left.

It's worth pointing out that some residents in dementia care units can still read. If we become more aware of this, we can greatly expand their activities and bring more meaning and enjoyment to their lives.

A New Vision of Dementia Care

Now that medical evidence has validated our decades-held belief that there is a "person" inside the individual with dementia—who may be functioning at a higher level than we think—we need a different way to relate to this individual. With Alzheimer's disease, the long-term memory stays intact the longest; the short-term memory fades away quickly. As a result, the individual will lose his or her recent memories while an experience from earlier in life remains intact for a long period of time. One of the unique traits of Alzheimer's disease is called "retrogenesis," which basically means that the person is mentally traveling backward in time. Based on the pioneering work of Dr. Barry Reisberg, retrogenesis involves mental abilities being lost as one gets older in the opposite order in which they were acquired during childhood. Reisberg and his team developed an assessment tool in the early 1980s called The Global Deterioration Scale (GDS) that documented how memories from adolescence and childhood appear to remain with the individual the longest. As Reisberg's work shows, it's our responsibility to find ways to "connect" through experiences the individual with dementia had in his or her formative years.

How can we begin to connect if we know nothing about the individual? First, we need to gather insights into the unique experiences the individual has had that hold a special place in his or her life. I firmly believe that you can't have a caregiving model focusing on the person if you don't ask the right questions when you're conducting the initial personal assessment. Holistic assessments are critical when an individual enters a dementia care unit. It's important to not only document the person's medical needs, but also the psycho/social components that can get short-changed in the admission process. Often, pieces of the assessment get divided up, with the social worker receiving one piece, the recreation director receiving another, and the nurse yet another. But if we have person-centered care, then why are vital aspects of the individual so divided up? Can we have a holistic view of the person when the critical pieces of information we must have to validate his or her needs are scattered? Absolutely not!

This brings me back, again, to Buddha's observation that "you cannot travel the path until you have become the path itself." While it's important we know everything we can about a person's past experiences, it's also important we understand what that person is experiencing under current circumstances. In the seminars I lead, I have attendees wear special glasses that simulate the visual experience of impairments such as glaucoma, cataracts, and macular degeneration. I also use auditory simulations to evoke feelings of anxiety, agitation and confusion. This is one simple way to experience what individuals with dementia may be experiencing; unfortunately, there's no way we can know for certain what they're actually feeling.

I read an article in the *New York Times* in which a medical student at the University of New England spent 10 days living in a nursing home.(8) The student was given a "diagnosis" of a particular ailment and was expected to live in the facility as someone with a similar condition. As a result, she experienced what she called an "emotional roller coaster," often feeling lonely and depressed. It was an eye opener for the student, and it should act as a wake-up call for everyone.

Until we've experienced these types of obstacles, how can we identify with these individuals' fears and apprehensions? How can we come closer to understanding their entire states of being and experiences?

I know how focused we as healthcare professionals can become on completing the task at hand, whether it's administering medications, carrying out the doctor's orders or maintaining shift coverage. It's not always easy to think about the person in front of you in addition to the task you have to perform, but it's vital to first consider the person's needs.

Maya Angelou said it best: "*We do what we have learned until we learn that what we do can be done a better way.*" In other words, we need to embrace change, not fear it. Instead, we need to fear remaining the same: by remaining static, we're not evolving. Yet life as we know it constantly evolves, with each moment presenting a new learning experience.

What we need to do is establish new roles for caregivers that embrace positive change. Once those new roles are clearly articulated by the employer and supported with the proper training, changes will begin to take place.

The following case study involving an Oregon assisted living facility provides an excellent example of what can be accomplished once we change the culture, and shows that change doesn't have to take years to implement.

Case Study: Jefferson Manor

In July of 2002, Jefferson Manor was a 70–bed facility with an occupancy rate below 50 percent. Faced with 41 pages of deficiencies and citations from the State of Oregon, the assisted living facility was on the verge of closure when a health care consultant for the states of California, Oregon and Washington assessed the situation.[9]

The consultant recommended new management and technology systems to restore the quality of care. Her recommendation meant significant changes had to be made—but if implemented quickly and correctly, it also meant the 36 residents who called Jefferson Manor home would not be displaced. A new management team was quickly assembled, and Vigilan, Inc., a provider of assisted living operations management systems, was brought on board. Within a week, the team developed an action plan that ensured regulatory compliance, consisting of new systems to continuously improve the quality of care and a new set of financial controls. The state accepted the plan with the caveat that the changes take place immediately. Measurable improvements had to be shown within 60 days.

Talk about changing the culture—and fast!

The facility's management conducted a residential and staff satisfaction survey that showed problems with the management staff. Appropriate staff-to-resident ratios were nonexistent, employees were unclear about their job responsibilities, and new employees received no mandatory training or orientation. All employees ended up needing to re-apply for their jobs due to this survey, which showed that the facility was serious about introducing changes, and enabling proper background checks to be conducted. This resulted in one-third of the staff being replaced. In addition, 40 hours of annual, mandatory training was implemented, which immediately raised morale and instilled confidence in the skills of the staff. As a result, the staff became friendlier and more cognizant of the residents' needs, and the residents responded in a positive manner, which helped to create a sense of community.

Jefferson Manor was also sorely lacking in processes and procedures, resulting in levels of care that were uneven at best and impossible to track. There was no system for managing medication delivery, no process for preparing and delivering nutritional food, and poor procurement procedures for supplies. A new operational management system from Vigilan was implemented, consisting of software that organized and connected resident assessments, care plans, staff assignments and billing.

The result? In just 60 days, the state conducted a comprehensive follow-up survey and found Jefferson Manor to be in "substantial compliance." Virtually every deficiency cited in the state's 41–page report had been eliminated. In the ensuing months, procedures were instituted requiring all new staff to receive initial training before interacting with residents; every employee received care and process training every two weeks and "just in time" training to correct performance issues on the spot.

Jefferson Manor was able to develop a culture of excellence in a relatively short period of time. In less than a year, it was able to make the transition from being potentially shut down to being recognized as one of the most advanced dementia care centers in the U.S.

Chapter 2
Beginning the Process of Transformation

As caregivers, we must lead the way. Sometimes, it seems that we are on a dimly-lit path—we can see the end, but we don't have enough illumination to get us there efficiently or effectively. This book was designed to provide you with practical advice that will help illuminate your path. Now, it's time to begin the process of transforming the culture.

A Change Is Going to Come

First, we must drastically modify the educational system for caregivers. It's as simple as that. If nursing assistant training included more information about how to better communicate with residents who have dementia, for example, then it might be possible to establish common bonds earlier. This training should start with basic information so the nursing assistant fundamentally understands how a person's brain functions are affected by the onset of dementia. This would help the assistant to better realize what a debilitating effect the disease has on an individual—and realize that the person's behaviors are not intentional.

Staff members want to provide care with the best of intentions, but they often can't tell if a person with dementia can comprehend what they're saying. That is why we need to give caregivers guidance and training about how to engage with a person on his or her level, taking into account the effects dementia has had on the individual. It's critical to have in-depth personal histories to serve this purpose which holistically focuses on the individual's life. Later in this book, I'll discuss the importance of using "conversation starters" as a means to engage with the individual, a list of potential conversation starters is included (*See* **Addendum A**).

Often, we feel like we're thrown into a job with a lot of procedural knowledge, but have little knowledge about the people under our care. If we want to transform our dementia care model, the first place to start is by changing the role of a caregiver into a "care partner". Second, we have to be sure to follow that education with effective training. And by effective, I mean training that is not only supported, but mandated.

The National Center for Assisted Living in 2010 compiled a state-by-state comparison of assisted living regulations which shows that states vary widely in terms of the regulatory control they exert over assisted living facilities that care for individuals with Alzheimer's disease or other types of dementia.(10) In some states, staff working in facilities with special care units must receive extensive initial training, usually within the first few months of employment, and then obtain continuing education credits. In other states, however, little if any initial training or continuing education is required. How this type of training can vary so much from state to state is bewildering, as formalized training can only benefit both the caregiver and the resident.

Finally, our systems and processes at long-term care facilities must change. We can't expect people with dementia to follow the same rules as those without dementia. For example, facilities need to curb the use of loud in-room paging systems; they are not only jarring, but they can also lead residents to think they're hearing voices. Another example: You may have a care unit where a nursing assistant is expected to get six to 10 residents up and dressed by 8 a.m. If even one of these individuals has dementia, this becomes a formidable task—for both the worker and resident. Supervisors will often talk with staff about the need to get the work done quickly and efficiently, but they seldom tell them how to get this done because it often cannot be done.

Consider two examples involving basic sleep patterns. Sleeping at night may be something most of us take for granted, but in the following examples, Frank's and Sandra's experiences show that their sleep patterns were based on the jobs they performed most of their lives.

Personal Example: Frank

Frank is 85 years old and has been told he has to be in bed by 7 p.m. like all the other residents. Well, Frank only needs seven hours of sleep, so he wakes up every day at 3 a.m. and walks the facility. He is tagged "the wanderer" and is given sleep medication. Unfortunately, the medication works all too well; after being awoken a few hours later, he's groggy while trying to get dressed in the morning. That leads to frequent falls as well as aggressive behaviors when he's forced to get up against his will. He's then medicated, again, to curb his aggressive behavior. As a result, the symptoms he's experienced due to dementia become exacerbated.

A look at Frank's personal history showed that he ran a bakery most of his adult life. Having to get up in the wee hours of the morning was part of his daily routine so the bakery cases could be filled with fresh-baked goods for the early-morning rush.

The upshot is that much of this could have all been avoided by a simple systemic change: allow Frank to go to bed at a later hour. This way, he'll get a good night's sleep and won't be up in the middle of the night.

Personal Example: Sandra

Similar to the example with Frank, Sandra is told she needs to be in bed by a certain time. Well, Sandra worked as a night nurse until she was 73 years old. Because of her schedule, she slept for a few hours in the morning, and then was up early in the afternoon to do her food shopping and visit with friends. She would catch a few more hours of sleep in the late afternoon/early evening before reporting for her shift. This had been her life since she was 25. So is it any wonder that Sandra wants to catnap during the day? Would it be that difficult to let her do that, then let her watch TV when she's up for a few hours during the middle of the night? Or switch her sleep schedule altogether so she can sleep during the day? Why must we feel like we're "warehousing" people to meet our criteria?

These examples are key to understanding how an individual's personal history can influence the way they act today, and why it's critical to have that historical information at your disposal.

When you think about it, none of the steps I've mentioned—education, training and system changes—is as difficult as rocket science. But these simple steps, taken together and implemented wisely, can lead to radical changes in the way we treat people with dementia.

Chapter 3

Improving the Quality of Life for People with Dementia

Having established the need for change relative to dementia training and education—and having shown how the simplest systemic changes can positively influence the individual—we need next to look at the importance of maintaining a person's quality of life. A person's quality of life is akin to their general well being. We know what makes our own quality of life rewarding; we also know what aspects of our daily lives tend to enrich us the most. What we need to do—what I will advocate through this book—is to ensure that individuals with dementia continue to perceive their lives to be meaningful for as long as they live.

For individuals with dementia, researchers have found that their quality of life depends on four things:

- The relationships they have with their family, their caregivers and other residents
- The level of control they have over their lives
- The way they spend their days, in terms of what they do and how they engage
- The ability to feel at home in their surroundings and feel safe, secure and comfortable

For us as caregivers, the key to providing a suitable quality of life is to find out what we can do to enhance the lives of others. By heightening our own awareness of what brings meaning and purpose to people whom we care for, we can act with the best intentions. This forms the basis for an approach I firmly believe in, which is called "intentional caregiving." Intentional caregiving simply means knowing what we're doing and why we're doing it.

What I find far too often is that caregiving tends to be done by rote. By rote, I mean the textbook dictionary definition: "from memory, without thought of the meaning; in a mechanical way."

But when we talk about care provided by a dementia care unit, we need to have an understanding of the "why' and "what." Why is the care provided by this unit so special? What is the unit doing to ensure its residents enjoy the best possible quality of life? These questions are only the start, but they provide the impetus for the cultural change on which we're embarking.

Building Relationships

Let's look at relationships and ask ourselves some simple questions: How do we form relationships? How do we build strong ones? How do we get to really know a person? How do we sustain a relationship built on trust with a person who has no memory?

It's important we begin by "getting to know" the people we care for as individuals. A good place to start is with a snippet of the lyrics from Rogers and Hammerstein's *The King and I*, a piece of music I use during the training sessions I conduct to illustrate my point:

> Getting to know you,
> Getting to know all about you.
> Getting to like you,
> Getting to hope you like me.
>
> Getting to know you,
> Getting to feel free and easy
> When I am with you,
> Getting to know what to say.

These lyrics were written from the point of view of a young woman who struck up a relationship with the children and the wives of the King of Siam. But I relate to the lyrics differently. In the context of dementia, the more we get to know about an individual with this disease, the better we can relate to the person, the better we can understand the behaviors that may be unique to him or her, and the better we can help to create a comfortable, secure and caring environment. As a result, these individuals will feel better about themselves when their needs are understood and met.

Under the new vision of dementia care I'm advocating, we need to get to truly know—and establish a vital communications link with—the individual inside the body of a person with dementia. I cannot overemphasize the fact that dementia profoundly impairs a person's ability to communicate effectively. Later in this chapter, you'll see how knowing pertinent facts about two residents' backgrounds made a huge improvement in their quality of life.

I've created a "Getting to Know You" personal history questionnaire that I encourage all families and facilities I work with to complete for the people within their care. To help you start creating this critical source of background information, I have listed a page of thought-provoking questions at the back of this book (*See* **Addendum B**).

In my consulting work, this is the first piece of information I review with caregivers. Most of the time, I find that histories collected are primarily based on medical information and omit the most important details about who the person actually is. This is something that long-term care facilities need to improve, because you can't market your facility as a specialized dementia care unit if your care is not "special." This type of initial background information must be unique to the individual and tell the person's whole story.

Granted, the admission process demands much from the attending family members. They may not be as focused on the personal aspect due to filling out many forms, including compiling the medical history. This can be confusing, exhausting and overwhelming. That's why it's important for a facility's admissions staff to work with families to educate them about why this personal information is so critical. For staff, it can be their only real connection to the individual inside the person with dementia. It's critically important for family members to understand the important role they play in helping the staff make a connection with their loved one.

This personal information needs to be clearly summarized, then broadly utilized with all the dementia care team members. This information, emphatically, should not be written on a chart that no one may ever read again; that will not do. Later in this book, I'll talk a little more about how this information will be used. But for now, remember that it's a small—but extremely important—step on our path toward effecting change.

Simply put, how we see a person influences how we provide for his or her care. If we view a person as a patient with behaviors, cognitive problems and physical complications, then we will treat this individual as a patient. But if we view the person as a human being, with a story to share and a life that's filled with memories and experiences, then we will treat him or her as a person just like us—who has a past, a present and a future.

The following examples from people I've worked with over the years demonstrate the important roles personal histories can play in getting to know the "person."

Personal Example: Raymond

Raymond lived in an extended care facility and was known for having a strong affinity for wooden furniture. He would go from table to table in the dining room, running his fingers across the edges of all the wooden surfaces, rubbing the flat surfaces with his hands. This behavior annoyed the staff; just when they had finished cleaning off a table, here was Raymond again, touching all the surfaces. Well, it turns out that he had been a furniture maker all his life. Once they found this out from his son, the staff began to appreciate Raymond due to the craft he'd practiced all those years. They even would ask him if the edges were mitered correctly when he was inspecting a dining room surface. Just think: they would have missed an opportunity to make Raymond feel special if they hadn't had that background about him and the sensitivity they developed as a result.

Personal Example: Bob

I once worked in a long-term care facility where Bob lived. He would routinely say, "I've got to get going—I'm going to miss my appointment!" Bob always seemed in a hurry to be going somewhere. Finally, I asked him, "Where do you need to go?" And he said, "Well, I've got a concert and I've got to get going!" It turns out that he'd played the banjo all his life and also played the harmonica. Nobody who worked at the long-term care facility knew that, and to this day I don't know why. Once we looked up his personal history and learned about his talent, we invited Bob to perform "concerts" regularly for the residents and their families to enjoy. We'd introduce him, he'd take a bow, and he'd play for 15 minutes. We purchased a few harmonicas for Bob as well.

Now if we'd never found out about Bob's talent, those "concerts" would never have happened! Because he provided entertainment for his fellow residents, this gave him a sense of pride and belonging.

We have to listen to what individuals are saying, look for clues that can be substantiated through their personal histories, and initiate questions that will give us a better understanding of how we can satisfy their needs.

As I've said, personal histories compiled upon admission to long-term facilities unfortunately aren't often shared as widely, or internally, as they should be. (Imagine how much Raymond and Bob's quality of life was enriched once their caregivers knew the reasons behind their actions.) This information should be readily available to all of the facility staff. It can be as simple as posting the information on the inside of every resident's closet. That way, if I'm taking care of someone, I'd know exactly where to look to find out more about him or her. A caregiver shouldn't have to dig to get this kind of crucial information.

Chapter 4
Building a Bridge to Better Care
Starts with the Caregiver

We've talked a bit about the need for understanding the individual. Now I'd like to turn to another type of relationship: the bonds between caregivers. I cannot overemphasize the importance of building a bridge between the individual, his or her family members, and the caregiver to ensure a quality of life that's worth living.

I firmly believe staff members who work in caregiving facilities need to become more familiar with each other. I do much of my work with hospitals, long-term care facilities, dementia units and adult day-care centers, so I know what types of training works best from firsthand experience. When I visit these facilities to lead training sessions, I begin by having each employee partner with another employee from a different department. Their task is to find commonalities they share by asking basic "Getting to Know You" questions. Facilities can do this with their own staffs by using the questions I've provided in the back of this book (*See* **Addendum B)**. The point is for coworkers to come to recognize each other as people in the truest sense of the word.

Staff Example: Amy and Pete

Take Pete and Amy, for example. They are coworkers at a long-term facility, where Pete is a dietary manager and Amy is a nursing assistant. Their goal is to come to know one another on a more personal level so they can establish a bond. That way, Amy is no longer simply "the nursing assistant" who works on the second floor;" instead, she's Amy, who graduated from the same high school Pete attended and has two younger brothers. And Pete is no longer just "the person who creates the residents' meals;" Amy finds out that he's a dog lover who shares her love for golden retrievers.

By establishing this concept of "getting to know you" among the staff first, it can then be applied in practice with the residents. Let's take this concept one step further to illustrate my point: what Amy has learned about Pete will help her as she forges a relationship with Mrs. Jones in Room 230.

Amy intentionally sets out to build a better relationship with the people she cares for. It begins with a simple, "You look comfortable today, Mrs. Jones." Amy then introduces herself by name and extends her hand. Mrs. Jones is pleased by the attention, and tells Amy to call her by her first name, Ida. After a while, Amy begins to relate to Mrs. Jones as Ida, a retired public school teacher who grew up in the same part of the Bronx as her grandmother.

Once Amy gets to know more about Ida, she understands why she likes her coffee piping hot: she always feels cold, no matter how many layers of clothes she wears. Amy tells this to Pete, who's in charge of the kitchen and tells his workers to put Ida's coffee on the dietary cart last, so it's as hot as can be when it reaches her. Amy takes this one step further by physically introducing Pete to Ida, making a true connection.

Staff Example: Luis and Maria

Here's another example that further illustrates my point: Luis from Maintenance is paired with Maria from Admissions to get to know each other better. They find that they are both from Portugal and both speak Portuguese fluently. As Maria finds someone with whom she can share conversations in her native language, she and Luis establish a common connection that transcends their job titles and roles. Later, Maria sits with a resident's family to discuss and document their "Getting to Know You" personal history about their father, Pasquale. His favorite vacation destination comes up in conversation, and Maria learns that he, too, is from Portugal! The conversation becomes personal, the connection deepens, and his family members now know that Maria will play an essential role on their father's caregiving team. After the meeting, Maria can't wait to tell Louis about Pasquale's arrival in their facility. Upon learning of this man's love for Portugal, Louis becomes a regular visitor, regaling Pasquale with stories about his heritage and establishing a connection.

It's not difficult, but it's how you start a cultural transformation: Relationships need to be established on a true, humanistic level. By taking small steps to familiarize the staff with each other, then applying that way of thinking to the facility's residents, common ground can be established. Suddenly you begin to see human traits you never took the time to notice in the past; on a deeper level, you begin to relate to people differently.

The same concept of relationship building can then be applied with a resident's family members. In Pasquale's case, the relationship was solidified when Maria offered up that she was from Portugal and shared a common heritage. Now Pasquale's family knows of at least one person they can contact if they have a question about their father's care. In Ida's case, Amy's nursing supervisor has taken it upon herself to get to know Ida's daughter a bit more. Due to Ida's chronic condition, the supervisor knows she will be in constant contact with her daughter. The next time she calls to inquire about her mother's condition, the daughter finds out that the nursing supervisor's teenage daughter is also getting ready to move away to college. Now, when the two of them talk about Ida, they start off asking each other how their daughter's college experience is turning out. There's another positive change: no longer is the facility only calling Ida's daughter when she suffers a setback. The nursing supervisor knows how much pressure Ida's daughter is under with the life changes taking place in her family and makes a point of calling her regularly when Ida has an exceptionally good day.

When I think about it now, I believe that Rogers and Hammerstein knew they had stumbled upon a good thing when they wrote "Getting to Know You" into the score of *The King and I* back in 1951. Now it's our turn to embed this way of thinking about relationships into our everyday lives, because it's one way to ensure that the dementia care we provide hits all the right notes.

Relationships Without Limitations Are Vital

In the past, caregivers were taught not to care too much—nor get too close—because developing such relationships with patients and family members was considered "unprofessional." (Yes, we were actually taught to keep our emotional distance!) In our new culture, however, the opposite is true. We need to make connections so we all are equal. It's what makes us human. This is why I often refer to the caregiver as a "care partner." When we are partners, we are two individuals working together toward a common goal. As partners, we learn about caring, kindness, listening, communication and, most of all, trust. We learn to respect the needs of the other individual and, together, we are seen as two equals. It is a reciprocal relationship—one where we benefit from the gifts we both give and receive.

This partnership philosophy must be woven into the fabric of each facility's building, organization and mission. It's not simply words but actions that we take to heart in our work every day. We need to build partnerships with each other, regardless of our title or role: staff with staff, staff with families, and staff with residents, residents with residents and residents with families; and yes, even families with families. Best-selling author Stephen Covey, a leadership expert, maintains that you always need to see the end in sight in order to know what you want to achieve.

If we practice what Covey prescribes, then our mission becomes clear. In order to provide the highest quality of care for people with dementia, we need to define the level of care required, specify what the end state should look like and begin to live the process by which we will get there. We need to strip away things that don't support and honor the person and rebuild from there. Does it happen overnight? Of course not! But we need to learn from what has not worked, break down the barriers that keep us separate, and rebuild from there.

Every Act of Creation Is First an Act of Destruction

You may be asking: Why destroy or change a system that has been in place for so many years? The answer is simply because the system is not working. We know this by examining what we've done in the past and still continue to do today. For example, how many medications are used for behaviors, sleep, agitation and aggressiveness? How many incidents and accidents occur between staff and residents, and between residents and residents? How often do staff members call in sick because of the stress on the job? Why is the turnover on the dementia care unit the highest of all units in healthcare facilities?

It's a fact that 90 percent of all behaviors are non-medical in nature, so this tells us that our practices need to change. Think about it: How often do we respond to families with a phrase like, "Well, that's the way our system works." How can we build a sense of trust with our employees, residents and families if our systems don't work and we continue to act as if everything is fine?

As we learn more about each other as people, the walls of separation begin to break down. With education and proper training, we can build character and competence among staff. This enables us to see all of the departments in an organization as part of a true team. We can also see the bigger picture of how residents, caregivers and families function together. Every team member in every department is vital to the success of our mission.

What we need to do is view these behaviors through a different lens. By viewing them as the result of unmet needs and broken systems, we can develop systems that offer opportunities to grow and provide the impetus for change for a better tomorrow. Let's delve into this further in the next chapter.

Chapter 5
Understanding What Behaviors Are Telling Us

With the background information in place—in other words, the "Getting to Know You Questions" completed and readily accessible by caregivers—we can better understand what a person's behaviors are telling us. But first, we need to start by understanding more about what constitutes an actual "behavior."

By definition, a behavior is simply a form of communication. It's the way we act or react to a situation and can be both verbal and non-verbal in nature. As we've discussed, dementia severely impairs a person's ability to communicate effectively and feel in control. Because of how the disease impacts the brain and its functions, a person's ability to decode and understand information is drastically diminished over time. That affects the individual's cognitive ability to put into words what he or she wants to say, as well as the individual's physical ability to actually get the words out. These language deficits are further compounded by other dementia-related impairments, such as memory loss, decreased attention span and impaired judgment. In effect, the person's ability to control how he or she thinks, reasons and acts becomes diminished.

As a result, we need a better understanding of how:

- Non-verbal behaviors are expressed by individuals with dementia
- Behaviors can be linked to the life history of a person
- Labels can actually harm a person with dementia whether we know it or not
- Descriptive observation and creative solutions can help a person with dementia feel understood
- Caregivers' behaviors affect a person with dementia

Non-verbal behaviors—which staff members sometimes interpret as agitation, restlessness, aggression and combativeness—are often expressions of unmet needs resulting from such causes as pain, discomfort, depression, sadness, loneliness or hunger. As you can tell from that description, there can be causes for a particular person's behavior. And just as importantly, there are many other ways people are telling us there's something wrong. They pace. They bang. They push. They shove. They grab. And yes, they even hit. Clearly when people act out physically or verbally, they're not happy. Then why sometimes do we ignore them? I often hear caregivers say, "Oh, they always do that." But the questions they should be asking themselves are, "Why are they doing that?" "What are their needs that we're not meeting?" "Do we even realize it when they are truly content, happy, and feeling good?" "What kind of behavior results when they're happy?"

It's critical to remember that people's impairments are a result of the disease and not—by any means—intentional behaviors on the part of the individual. This can be difficult for untrained caregivers to accept and deal with, demonstrating why a new way to train and educate staff is essential if we want to share a common vision of change.

One of the most common behaviors we observe when people are newly admitted to long-term care facilities is an overwhelming desire to leave the building. They desperately want to find a way out in order to go home; inside, they are frantic, trying to figure out what has happened to their world. This is when people feel their control is slipping away. Behaviors can run the gamut of emotions: from fear and tears, to yelling and screaming, to anger and depression. Many times persons with dementia will experience the exact same emotions you or I would have in a similar situation. Their perception may be different, but the emotional response may be exactly the same.

What we fail to recognize when dealing with people with dementia is that we all need to have a purpose in life. Once our purpose in life—whatever it may be—is taken from us, we simply don't know what to do with ourselves. You or I may take this for granted during the course of our typical workday, but think about how people feel when they retire. A big adjustment is in order, because recent retirees no longer have their regular daily routines. Their sense of purpose is lost. They may start to lose a sense of who they really are as if they were inextricably tied to their career or job. Now take this one step further, and think about how individuals with dementia feel when they are removed from all they know that's familiar. It's unsettling, to say the least.

Adjusting to Change

I'd like you to take a moment and think about how you would feel if, after living in your home for 40 years, you were whisked away from the place you were most familiar with. How would your behavior change if you were left with few possessions, an unfamiliar bedroom, a roommate who you did not know and a building filled with strangers? In a place where nothing felt familiar, you certainly wouldn't be comfortable, would you? It's important to think about what emotions and behavior you would exhibit upon being told that you no longer had control over where you were going to live.

This would undoubtedly raise some questions on your part, wouldn't it? "Am I ever going home?" "What happened to my home and all my things?" "Whom am I living with?" "What happened to my pet?" "Where is this place?" "Will I ever see my family and friends again?" "How will I get to church?" "What happened to all my money?" "Did I do something bad to deserve this?"

Even if you didn't have dementia, think about how you would feel upon hearing that news: you'd feel frustrated, angry, annoyed, and probably frightened out of your mind. Now think about how your behavior might change if you had to do this against your will. If you lost control of every aspect of your life, wouldn't that be a major challenge?

Now think back to what I was saying earlier about how our quality of life depends on the relationships we have and our ability to exhibit control over our lives. Clearly, in this type of situation, a person will have to form all-new relationships. And control?—clearly any sense of control is gone.

Now think about what happens when a person in our care exhibits negative behaviors. What do we do? Instead of trying to understand what he or she may be feeling, we may resort to labeling this person as "challenging" or "difficult." This person has just been uprooted from home, and everything held dear for an entire lifetime has been taken away—yet we're annoyed because the individual is resistant to change? Or worse, because it's messing up our schedule?

Why is it that when residents seem not to be following our rules or living up to our expectations, we get frustrated and place labels on them? These individuals are not necessarily resisting our care; instead, they are reacting to their loss of control by resisting the regimentation we impose on every aspect of their lives. Can't we see that?

Labels are hurtful. Labels dehumanize the person. We don't see Mary or John as people once they are labeled; we see them as the hitter, the biter or the kicker. In seminars I've led, I've heard more labels than I care to admit: Houdini, the wanderer, the grabber, the walkie-talkie, the left fielder, the right fielder... the list goes on and on. Labels are still being applied because individuals fail to conform to the "norm." But what is the "norm" when we're talking about something as ambiguous as Alzheimer's disease? When we talk about a change in the culture for dementia care, we need to start by focusing on the whole individual—not a one-dimensional label applied in haste, ignorance and frustration.

Again, this is why the need for education and training is so important—to help us see the person inside the façade clouded by dementia. By applying labels, we're dehumanizing the individual.

Staff Example: Sally and Rita

I observed an example of how a person can be instantly dehumanized when I was working in a long-term care facility not that long ago. Two of the nursing assistants, Sally and Rita, got into a screaming match with one another. This took place in a resident's room. The resident could not speak, and I'll never forget the look of fright on her face. Sally and Rita stopped their heated argument as soon as I entered the room, but I fear that it wouldn't have stopped soon otherwise.

I use this example to ask the following question: "Would these two staff members have carried on so vehemently if the person in their presence was cognitively intact?" I seriously doubt it! Sadly, the perception was that this person could not hear, speak, or understand. I'm sure these caregivers were thinking, "She's demented—she doesn't know what's going on."

When Sally and Rita tried to give physical care to this individual right after this incident, the resident's kicking and grabbing was most certainly a result of the fear she had just experienced. The point to take away from this scenario is sad but true: the caregivers did not see this person as a human being with feelings; they saw her as someone who was demented. As a result, they couldn't even see how their argument had upset and affected her.

Unfortunately, if untrained staff members view a person as demented and unable to express his or her needs, they can perceive this person to be less human than they are. This clearly reinforces the need for specialized classes and follow-up training.

Chapter 6
The Relationship Between Behaviors and Routines

Individuals with dementia for whom "specialized" care units have been created will have the most difficulty with routines surrounding their personal care. These routines are highly regimented so the facility can smoothly operate. Typically, these routines were created to accommodate internal processes, staffing schedules and employee work flows. But what about the individuals requiring care? Why aren't the routines created around their likes and dislikes?

This is the primary reason why a Dementia Care Unit needs to institute a policy that states, "We are here to serve our residents." And what exactly does this mean, you may ask? It means you don't need to get each and every resident up at a certain time if they don't want to! It means that care needs to be personalized based upon their life-long routines—and it means that our 7-3, 3-11, and 11-7 world needs to be revamped.

Again, we need to take a look at the residents' histories. There may be underlying reasons—based on an individual's daily routine before the onset of dementia—that show why a prescribed routine simply won't work.

The Need for Respect

I won't argue that getting people dressed sometime during the day is an important goal. But it's just as important for us to learn to respect a person's individual routine. When you think of your morning routine—and how it's sequenced—you'll see why people with dementia are used to the daily routines they've followed for years. We have to respect that and sympathize with why they're finding it difficult to adapt to "our" routine.

Think, for a moment, about everything we're asking individuals with dementia to do, and how it would feel if we were faced with these orders. It would be odd for me, for example, to wash my back before I washed my face in the morning. If someone were washing my back and then started to wash my feet against my will, I might kick them to make them stop.

Yet when we're bathing residents or giving any physical care, we often do have a set routine we follow. It's the way we train staff so they can get their work done in the most efficient way. However, we need to realize that our routine may not be the resident's routine, and we need to find ways to better relate to the individual's daily needs and routines.

This gets back to what I was saying about knowing as much as we can about a person's habits and routines. Lanny Butler wrote a wonderful book called "My Past Is Now My Future" that I highly recommend. What we perceive to be true for ourselves often becomes the reality we assume for others, his book asserts. In other words, just because we eat, bathe and sleep at certain times in certain ways doesn't mean people with dementia will want to change their personal habits to accommodate ours.

I realize there may be a fine line between perceived neglect and intentional caregiving. Appearances can often be misleading. Checks and balances need to be in place, most certainly. And yes, we have to be communicating not only with each other but also with family members so they, too, understand the rationale behind changes they see in regular routines. We have to assure them that proper care will be given so they'll understand why, if they come to visit in the afternoon, their mother might still be in her nightgown. Having established a bond with the family, as I mentioned earlier, will serve us well when we're trying to change the culture by focusing on the residents' individual needs. When families are part of the new culture, they understand what we're doing, why we're doing it, and how their family member will benefit from it. They will begin to place their trust not only in you, but also in the process as well.

There are four simple words that form the basis of a question I ask in these types of scenarios: "How important is it?" For example, if dressing someone is causing a catastrophic reaction, we need to ask ourselves, "How important is it to get him or her dressed at that moment?"

Now that we know there's a strong relationship between routines and behaviors, let's look at a few examples that show how a resident's needs are very similar to our own.

Personal Example: Betty

Betty was labeled by her caregivers as "the screamer" and "the nail digger." Every day when she was given her shower, her cries from the bathroom were excruciating. I observed the staff interacting with her, both before and during the shower. Actually, there was very little interaction, with little if any conversation taking place on a personal level. The conversation between the caregivers and Betty was mainly instructional. So, once the water was turned on, the screaming started. The staff followed a regimented routine: first, Betty was seated in a shower chair. The water would then come down on her back and hair first, and staff would begin by washing her hair. Betty would hold her hands close to her body, as if she was protecting her chest. Following the shower, the screaming would continue, with Betty being inconsolable for most of the day.

Looking at historical information about Betty's life, it was clear that she always took showers, but never—*ever*—washed her own hair in the shower. Betty routinely went to the beauty parlor weekly to have her long hair washed and set. I surmised that Betty was getting upset during the regimented routine because it was so different from what she had experienced in the past.

When I talked with Betty's daughter, I found out that she never liked the cold weather and lived in Florida until she came to this particular facility in New York. Finding out more about Betty and her daily routines helped us to revise how care would take place. We connected her with a caregiver who was originally from Florida herself and loved the hot weather. This particular caregiver enjoyed classical music as much as did Betty and shared her passion for growing orchids, which Betty did upon her retirement. In fact we learned that Betty had won many top prizes for her orchids in flower shows.

Betty's story is a prime example of why looking into the personal history and habits of an individual can give us the clues we need to dramatically improve her quality of life. It may not always go perfectly, but by trying, exploring and creating, we can learn a great deal. As I said in the beginning of this book, it requires taking the time to walk in a person's shoes to gain insight into their habits and behaviors.

Here's how Betty's situation was turned around. Staff members were trained in how to provide care under the new model for dementia care I promote in this book. They spent time talking with Betty before it was time for her to shower. The staff member I mentioned from Florida sometimes would bring in an orchid and talk to Betty about it for a few minutes. She would ask Betty for her opinions. How often should the orchid be watered? How often should it be fed? What nutrients should it be fed? They would share this connection, making it a meaningful engagement. Betty was offered a pink or blue shower cap to keep her hair dry and in place. We followed the routine of her past habits, washing her face first. We placed a terry wrap around her to keep her covered, especially since it was winter and colder than usual. The staff played soft classical music in the background during her shower. When the shower was over, the staff was amazed that Betty did not scream—not even once! Instead, Betty looked happy and content as she swayed to the music with a smile, and she seemed to look forward to the weekly shampoo and style at the beauty parlor.

Personal Example: Armand

Just as Betty was labeled, so was Armand. He was known as "the wanderer" and "the banger." I heard staff from one shift to the next warn each other to watch out for him. Here's why: Armand had a routine of waking up at 4:30 a.m. and banging on the unit's exit door with his fists. He did not speak, but his anger was most obvious through his constant pounding on the door. When he would start to get tired, he would take a break and walk in and out of other residents' rooms. But soon he would be back to the exit door and start pounding away again. How did the staff address the behavior? They would stay seated and yell, "Armand, stop it!" "Armand, don't go in that room!" "Armand, you can't go out!"

The first step in truly addressing the behavior and understanding its underlying causes was to get to know Armand through his personal history. Once the staff took the time to read up on Armand, they learned that he had owned a landscaping business for almost 40 years. He loved being outside—being one with nature—and always took a morning walk to see his plants, shrubs and landscape designs. This had been his routine for nearly all of his life. Since his business had always been in his family, his walks with his father at an early age were also part of his history. Armand spoke French and was raised in the little town of Lyon. He spoke English perfectly, but for the past seven years, he had not conversed verbally. He had entered the facility just six weeks prior, and the staff already wanted to medicate him to calm him down. When I asked his caregivers how often Armand was able to walk outdoors, the staff simply replied, "It's winter!"

The fact that staff applied labels to him upon his admittance to the facility exemplifies how a person can be dehumanized. I find it interesting that when you or I walk, we are usually walking with a purpose in mind. We may be going for a walk with someone, getting our daily exercise or making our way to a destination. But if we see a man with Alzheimer's disease walking around in circles, and it appears to us that he has no purpose, then he's labeled a "wanderer." I prefer to think of a person who wanders as someone who is looking for something; perhaps he or she just hasn't figured out what that "something" is! Maybe the person does know what they're looking for and we're just not aware of it. Again, we have to remember that an individual with dementia may never be able to tell us why he or she is behaving in a certain way.

So what became of Armand? He was simply taken outside each day—yes, even in the winter with a coat, shoes and a hat! After 10 minutes in the fresh air, he would sit comfortably in a chair and enjoy a cup of coffee with his caregiver. It was interesting to find out that the caregiver who took him on his morning walks was not even in the facility's nursing department. Joe was from the maintenance department. He spoke French, loved to garden and bonded with Armand very quickly. He had recently lost his own father, so his daily routine with Armand brought more meaning to his life as well. This is a good example of a connection that had great meaning and worth to both individuals.

I know you are probably reading this and saying to yourself, "How can we possibly do this?" I want to say, here and now, that if we continue to do what we have done in the past, nothing will change. Nothing! It takes leadership, a vision, a plan and a team of creative, caring people to make it work because they understand that everyone's lives need to have meaning.

Looking at behaviors from different perspectives is critical to changing a culture. I contend that true culture change begins with each and every employee—no matter what job, what level or what department. We need to relate to people with dementia as human beings and see what they represent beyond the challenges they possess. Remember: People are not their illnesses, nor are they their behaviors.

Chapter 7

The Effect of Pain on a Person's Behavior

It's important to remember there could be another reason why some residents won't do everything we want them to do or act out verbally or non-verbally. Simply put, they could be experiencing pain. These individuals could be experiencing some form of discomfort that dramatically affects their quality of life, and we don't even know it!

Every day, 70 million Americans are dealing with some sort of chronic pain. It's important to realize that the burden of chronic pain is greater than that of diabetes, heart disease and cancer combined. Yet most of the time, pain is not assessed for individuals with dementia. As a society, we tend to blame everything on dementia and take many things for granted. "They're biting, they're tugging—oh, it must be their dementia." But maybe it's that the person can't tell you the real reason is, "My body aches," or, "I'm really in a lot of pain when you do that." People may be experiencing discomfort or pain associated with such conditions as arthritis, past adhesions, constipation, headaches, sore knees or swollen ankles. Many of the residents under our care don't have the verbal skills necessary to tell us that. So, as a result, they act out behaviorally because they can't express their feelings or needs in any other way.

Let's look at some examples from my work to illustrate this point.

Personal Example: Sandra

Sandra was a resident who walked all the time. On this particular day, however, she was crying as she made her way down the corridor. She was not holding any particular part of her body, or tugging at anything. Her gait appeared the same as usual, a fast pace. But when the staff tried to remove her shoes for a nap, she screamed loudly. In order to appease her, they decided to let her keep her shoes on this time. Once she fell asleep, they removed her shoes and socks to find four toes badly bruised, swollen and fractured. It had never occurred to the nursing assistant that this was the problem, since the resident's pace and gait appeared normal.

Certified nursing assistants are the ones most apt to observe what's happening with the resident. But let's face it: they have hard jobs. That's why it's essential to teach them critical observational skills. They've been trained to do a job and complete a list of duties in a certain way. If they're busy completing those tasks, they're more focused on the job at hand rather than the actual human being. It's not their fault—it's the way they've been trained.

It's time to train our front line staff differently. They need to intentionally look into the resident's face to see what emotion is being felt. Staff also needs to be taught how residents' body movements are indicative of their physical comfort level—they must observe the way residents move their hands and fingers, for example, assessing each movement. They need to look at when a person may wince, cry, or move away. This is an observational skill that must be taught, practiced and considered a priority. This approach is essential for intentional caregiving.

Assessing Pain

It is important for us to remember that dementia does cause postural changes. We need to understand that there is damage to the motor cortex, which in turn affects a person's posture and gait. A person's stance will widen, for example; their knees bend more and their ability to walk normally is lost. A person begins to walk with a shuffled gait. Walking in this manner hurts, and postural changes can be uncomfortable and painful. The body pulling in this way causes added strain on the shoulders and back. If you have ever had a backache, can you imagine the discomfort a person with this condition can be in? We also need to consider the person who is in a wheelchair, unable to walk. What type of discomfort does being confined to a chair create? Could any one of us imagine being stuck in a chair, unable to get up and walk somewhere?

I remember reading a research paper that looked at the correlation between agitation, pain and scheduled doses of Tylenol. The study stated that when Tylenol was given around the clock, people had less agitation. This proved to decrease pain levels, thus reducing the incidence of agitation. Again, are some of the behaviors we see expressions of pain and discomfort?

Additionally, I'd be remiss if I didn't acknowledge the difficulty we have in health care of properly caring for people's teeth. Dental care is not being performed adequately for individuals with dementia—in fact, sometimes it's not being performed at all. A person could be experiencing a toothache, gum disease or poorly fitted dentures—all factors that could be causing his or her sudden change in behavior and may also be affecting the individual's appetite. But we can't tell that's the cause because the resident can't tell us! Is anyone monitoring the resident during meal time? Are we looking at facial expressions? Is the person holding a side of his or her mouth or pulling on his or her ear? Is someone refusing to eat because the person's gums and teeth are sensitive? The point I'm making is simple: we need to heighten our observational skills to better understand the role something as routine as dental care can play in affecting something as important as a person's ability to eat.

Personal Example: Ben

Ben would wake up every day at 3 a.m., when he would begin walking up and down the halls. He would pass the nurse's station, bang on the desk and then walk away. The staff would be instructed to put him back to bed, which they did, but within a few minutes the behavior would begin again. They finally got an order for sleeping medication that they administered at 4 a.m. The unfortunate part of this story is that at 6 a.m., he was wakened for his shower. That's when the battle would begin! As a result, he was labeled aggressive, combative and uncooperative. Is it any wonder?

Many times residents are placed in bed at 7 p.m., and after seven or eight hours of sleep they are ready to start their day. Ben was a perfect example. He simply had rested enough for what his body needed, so at 4 a.m. he was ready to start his day—and ready to let everyone know it. It turns out that he was being put to bed way too early for his body to adjust. Once again, our regimented systems didn't support the person. Once Ben was allowed to go to bed later, he would sleep until close to 6 a.m. and be more alert when he started his day.

Unfortunately for Ben, another instance occurred related to his behavior and discomfort. During one dining occasion, Ben refused to eat and was being overseen by a nursing assistant who was taken from another unit to help with breakfast. This nursing assistant was not given any history or pertinent information about Ben, but was simply instructed to help him with his meal. Ben refused to eat, and so she proceeded to assist him. Ben took one bite of his toast, started to yell and threw his tray on the floor. The nursing assistant reported this encounter as the resident was not hungry and he was very agitated. Later that same day, another caregiver who had worked with Ben before noted while helping him with mouth care that his gums were sore, swollen and extremely reddened. Ben was in pain, and the observation of his comfort was not consistent from one caregiver to another. Once again our system did not support the resident.

That's why finely-tuned observational skills are so important for the staff. In the back of this book (*See* **Addendum C**), you'll find a pain assessment form that can be used for this purpose. The form will help nursing assistants identify a movement or activity that causes an individual pain. This could be something as simple as brushing one's teeth—or something as complex as lifting the person out of bed. This simple sheet can be immensely helpful when we talk about a culture of intentional caregiving. In fact, I recommend that the sheet be used several times a day—a simple check and balance, if you will, to get the caregiver more attuned to observing and recording any noticeable cause of pain. It's critical for pain to be assessed on a regular basis—and for staff to be educated and trained on the proper use of observational techniques.

The pain assessment form is important, quite frankly, because our observational skills are often sorely lacking. By using the form during the course of the day, you'll be able to tell if a person hurts at a certain time of day. This also adds value to the role of the nursing assistant, and brings both the science and the art back to nursing. They can actually see how they're affecting an individual's life.

It's critically important for all staff on the dementia care team be trained and educated on how to assess pain. Every team member will come into contact with the resident in different settings. They need to be constantly observing those in their care. They also need to know what to do with this information. For example, many times people working in Housekeeping feel it's their job just to keep the rooms and unit clean. Individuals in Recreation may feel their goal is just to keep people engaged in meaningful activities. The Food and Nutrition staff may feel their job is just to prepare the food. But clearly, everyone's job is larger and greater than that! In the new dementia care culture, it is everyone's job on the team to care for the resident. We need to supply the education for this to happen, and change the scope of everyone's job to see the bigger picture.

Physical and Emotional Pain Is Under Treated

Earlier in my career, a resident fell at one of the facilities where I worked. When the resident and the nursing assistant got to the hospital, they were told she'd need sutures in her head. The intern said, "Well, we're just going to sew her up." The nursing assistant, who was trained in dementia care, thankfully, said "You're going to give her Novocain, aren't you?" And the intern said, "Nah—those people don't feel pain." Needless to say, the resident did receive Novocain and the proper medical treatment, but only because the nursing assistant was aware and spoke up.

I still read articles where people with dementia aren't being given pain medication during medical procedures because they don't ask for it. Unfortunately, this happens all the time. Nurses aren't

being trained—and doctors aren't being trained—and they're or-
dering medicine "PRN," which means whenever necessary. But if
people with dementia are unable to express themselves verbally,
and the attending physicians and nurses aren't watching them, they
aren't going to be receiving any pain medication!

In terms of understanding pain and discomfort, you'll have
individuals with dementia "act out" simply because it hurts. If
you've got arthritis, then just putting a shirt on over your head can
be extremely painful. Having someone lift your arms to put them
into a piece of clothing can feel like torture.

Clothing: the Need for a Perfect Fit

Clothing for people with dementia most certainly needs to be
examined closely. If their clothing is causing them discomfort—
if you see people wincing or yelling when you're getting them
dressed, for example—then they're very likely to be in pain. If
they even see you coming toward them, with their clothing in
your hands, they view this as a sign that you're going to hurt them.
Again, they won't be able to tell you, but they may show agitation
by simply wanting to protect themselves. That's a perfect example of why people might act out aggressively.

Clearly in a circumstance like this, the caregiver would never
intend to hurt the individual. But as I said at the beginning of this
book, intentional caregiving is all about placing the individual's
needs first, intentionally looking for ways to make the person's
quality of life as good as possible. In this case, a caregiver should
think about making accommodations to a patient's clothing, as
there are many ways to do this. You can take a shirt and put Velcro closures in the back, so a person doesn't have to lift his or her
arms to put it on. Or, instead of having something that needs to
be put on over someone's head, you can use a zipper or snaps to
make getting dressed as comfortable as possible.

We need to continually use our skills to assess if those under
our care are in pain, or if there are other reasons for the emotions

they're showing. They could be lonely, tired or depressed. While there are times that pain certainly needs to be treated, there are also times that someone may just need companionship. He or she might be crying, screaming, or yelling as a result of being lonely or bored.

This is why teaching observational skills for all team members is critical. If we see someone having discomfort during bathing, something as simple as giving them a dose of Tylenol 30 minutes before bath time may be all that's needed. While figuring this out can be complicated and confusing, it's part of what our role requires.

Showing people how to troubleshoot and creating personalized plans of care are key. To remind myself of this, I use the phrase, "Inspect what you expect." Then ask yourself the following questions:

- "Did the new treatment work?"
- "Did I give it ample time to work?"
- "Did I try a few different things?"
- "What worked, what didn't, and why?"

Personal Example: June

I remember when I was working in a facility and went to say hello to June, one of the residents. She immediately grabbed my hand and squeezed very hard, not wanting to let go. Her grip was very tight. I smiled and relaxed my hand so there was not a struggle. Many times when we are responding, our bodies will tighten up out of fear and we begin a struggle of force. One person tries to get out and the other person remains in control by squeezing even harder. I developed a program called "The Trusting Touch™" that gives caregivers steps they can use to respond with skill and knowledge in situations where they feel threatened or at risk.

In June's case, once I relaxed my fingers and sat down to talk with her, I felt her hand release. Our smiles connected, and we talked for a while. I wasn't really doing anything except offering a kind word or two. And then I continued with my work. Do we ever stop and ask ourselves to think about how an individual's world can shrink when he or she has this disease? Or how few meaningful interactions this person has each day?

Pain can be both physical and emotional, and we all need to do a better job of remembering that in our daily lives. We need to be cognizant of the fact that a person does not need to be visually expressing pain to be experiencing pain. We also need to remember the fact that pain not only has physical causes, but emotional origins as well. Once we have an understanding of why someone is in pain, we can start to think about what they need to treat the pain.

Integrative, Complementary Therapies and Treatments

We have to make sure that we don't immediately jump to giving people pain medication unnecessarily to treat a behavior. There is a fine line here because we know there could be increased falls or other complications. We have to think of the non-pharmacological measures, such as warm and cold compresses, therapeutic touch, hand or foot massage, reflexology and music that can help them relax and alleviate pain and discomfort. It's important to integrate different types of therapies wherever possible.

Here's a prime example: A recent Yale University study found that delirium in hospitalized elderly patients is common and often unrecognized, with the potential to lead to serious complications.[11] What these researchers did was to institute a protocol to reduce the risk of delirium. Here's how they did it: To avoid the use of sleeping medications (a leading risk factor for delirium), they developed a non-pharmacologic sleep protocol that could be implemented by the nursing staff or trained volunteers. Part of the protocol involves offering a back rub, warm milk, and soothing music to aid in relaxation. The result was profound: The Yale Delirium Prevention trial was the first trial to show that delirium can be prevented by instituting a night-time relaxation program to reduce the need for sleep medications.

Chapter 8
Learning How to Recognize the "Feeling" Tone

As I mentioned earlier, the ability for an individual to feel at home in his or her surroundings is tantamount to ensuring that a person's quality of life continues to be satisfying. That's why we need to do our best to give people what they need—both physically and emotionally—so they can feel safe, secure and comfortable.

Even if we don't understand what people are saying — even if it's indiscernible — we need to be sensitive to the "feeling tone" in their behaviors. In other words, the message is in the manner in which they're expressing their feelings. Only when we tune in to that message can we understand and deal with a person's true emotional state.

For example, when residents in your facility cry out over and over "mama mama ... mama mama ... mama mama," that might be because of feelings of fear and insecurity they feel in their present-day environment. They could be thinking about their mothers and expressing their longing to return to the safety and security of childhood years. We can usually determine the feeling tone that is at the root of such behavior if we take the time to watch and observe the residents closely. When we make the effort to look at inexplicable behaviors in this way, we become much better caregivers.

Unfortunately, what often happens is that we become so immune to our residents' "sense of being" that we walk right past them. We might hear someone on the unit say, "Just ignore her—she does that all the time." In fact, we need to do just the opposite. She could be banging on the table all the time because she likes the sound of the noise. In fact, it makes her feel alive—did you ever think of that? She hears a sound—and it's caused by something she's doing—and to her it feels like she's doing something. That's what we need to find out. We can't just walk away thinking that her behavior doesn't mean anything. When we do take pause and get down at her eye level and hold her hand, does the behavior stop? Is it that she wants attention? Is it that she's lonely? It's our job to look for what she's trying to communicate. She may not remember your name, but she will feel and remember your touch.

Personal Example: Catherine

Catherine was non-verbal and would scream when someone new tried to get her into bed from her wheelchair. But when one particular nurse came into the room, she would call Catherine by name, touch her hand and stroke her hair. Catherine would kiss her and let her put her into bed. Whether the pain is physical or emotional we need to stop, look, and listen!

As caregivers, we need to learn how to be there when somebody is frustrated, anxious or sad. We need to understand why this person is crying and why he or she is feeling this way. It's not enough to say, "Catherine, you should be happy—cheer up!" When we get sad, what do we need? We want to hear someone say, "I'm here for you—you're not alone." We don't want to feel that we're alone—we want someone to listen. Why should we expect any different from individuals with dementia? Why can't we allow them to express what they need to express? After all, we are their connection to life itself, and we could all use a little training in how to make that connection stronger. Again, that's why historical backgrounds are essential.

When we look at individual behaviors of self-expression, it's important to look at how our non-verbal communications—or our "approach"—can affect another person. A feeling tone certainly doesn't have to be verbal, as the example that follows will illustrate.

Staff Example: Elaine

At one facility where I worked, I watched Elaine, one of the nurses, pound pills with a pill crusher right in front of the resident. Even though this was a silent pill crusher, the intention was to get the pills to a consistency as fine as possible. Elaine also enjoyed getting out her frustrations doing this exercise. She made no eye contact with the resident, but put applesauce on a spoon with the grounded pills and said, "Take this." When the resident threw the cup on the floor, Elaine said, "Why did you do that?" She then marked her down on her chart as "non-compliant." Is it any wonder?

Wouldn't a smile, a soft touch, and a kind word have been better medicine than that pill the nurse was trying to have her take? Her actual eye contact and soft touch may have benefited that person more than the pill did. What was this resident's need? Was it the need to just feel human? Was it a need to feel important and valued? Was it a need arising from thirst or hunger? Did the pounding seem like a violent or angry action? Or was it that she simply had a headache from Elaine's pounding of the pills? As I've said before, every behavior means something.

This problem was easily resolved: Elaine became mindful that she needed to crush the pills without undue force. She also made some additional changes: she spoke with the resident before administering the medication and they spent a few moments together. They both liked pansies, so they admired the ones on the counter. Elaine then said, "I have something for you" and gently placed her hand on the spoon and helped to guide it into her mouth. Elaine then thanked her for the help she provided.

Some caregivers want to simply check off their list and get their work done as quickly as possible. Sure, their co-workers see them as fast and efficient. But how do their residents view them? Is the resident screaming, resisting, and pushing away?

It's not always just one thing in particular we can point to about why residents resist. But we need to put more thought into this: Are we rushing them just to get our work over with? Are we going too fast? Are we outpacing them? Are we making each encounter positive? Are we getting into their personal space too quickly?

Think About New Processes

In nursing, we usually follow a set process where we do something to the individual, such as distribute medication. I'm a strong believer in looking at every process we use to find ways to not only save time, but also spend more quality time with residents.

The process for distributing medication is a prime example: it's a labor-intensive activity that consumes a good portion of a caregiver's time—time that could be put to better use.

We need to start by asking ourselves, "Are there any medications we can eliminate such as vitamins and other supplements that aren't being absorbed anymore?" Another important question is: "Can't we avoid passing out meds at mealtimes so more time can be devoted to the meal itself?" According to the American Journal of Nursing, consolidating the distribution of medicine can lead to more free time to spend with patients.(12) At St. John's Home, a facility in Rochester, N.Y., the need for a 5 p.m. medication pass was eliminated altogether, and there was a reduction in the number of times per day—and per shift—that patients had to be given medications. Think about how much more time the caregivers there now have to spend with their residents.

I'm also a strong believer in doing periodic check-ins on our own behavior to find things we can change about ourselves that will have positive effect on those we care for. For example, our conversations should never be stressful; in fact, we should make every effort to let the person know that they're right. We can start that practice by eliminating the word "no"—and anything negative for that matter—from our vocabulary. When we say something like "Don't do that" or "Don't go in that room," we're using a negative tone whether we realize it or not. The resident will not only see it in our body language; he or she will see it in our facial expressions. All we're going to do is confuse the person. They may recognize that's something not right, but cognitively, they won't be able to figure it out.

Make Every Day Matter

It's important to make sure that every part of the day is great for someone with dementia. You want that positive feeling tone to resonate long after you've left the room. For example, instead of saying, "So, you have to eat more of your lunch today, Sadie," you change it around to say, "It looks like you're enjoying your lunch today, Sadie. Your lunch looks wonderful. I'm going to take a moment and have something to eat with you."

In other words, you wouldn't say, "What did you do all day?" Instead, you'd say, "You look like you had a nice day today, Sadie—I saw your drawings and they're beautiful." You want to ask basic "yes or no" questions. You want to keep it simple.

Remember: The last word you use in a sentence usually is the last one the person with dementia is going to hear. For example, if you say to someone, "Don't stand up!" What do they do? Stand up—because "up" is the word this person will hear. We've got to ensure that the way we communicate will be both positive and instill the meaning at the end of the sentence.

An individual with dementia will usually be able to comprehend three words out of a sentence. As the disease continues, it might deteriorate into two words... then one word. Most of the time caregivers use the word "okay" at the end of their sentence. Why is this wrong? Because the resident is likely to just repeat the word "okay," leading the caregiver to think that everything is fine when it might not be.

Some key things to remember:

- Yes/no questions generally work well
- Limit choices to two to make it easier for them to comprehend
- Remove the word "no" from your vocabulary at all costs
- Give compliments and make eye contact, because positive affirmations based on observations can leave a lasting impression

Many times we're instructed in our training to tell the residents everything we're going to do. That's fine if the residents have cognitive abilities. But someone with dementia will likely have difficulty processing the information in the way we are used to giving it. He or she is simply not going to understand.

The key is to simplify it and break it down step by step. I always talk about the "20-second" rule: it takes a minimum of 20 seconds for the person to be able to absorb information and process it. Normally we ask a lot more questions during those 20 seconds. If we stop, look at the person and time 20 seconds on our watch, it's going to feel like an eternity. Why? Because we are uncomfortable with silence! As caregivers, we feel like we've got to keep moving, fill the space, and move on. We have to learn to stop, pause and wait for a reaction.

Training Exercise: Reversing Roles

Here's a role playing exercise you can use to sensitize your staff: Put on soothing music and ask one employee to pretend to be the resident, and the other to play the caregiver role. Have the "caregiver" take the "resident's" hands in their hands and be instructed to make that other person feel safe. You want to make them feel that they are loved without saying any words. Usually, when I do this in my training sessions, the participants can barely last a few seconds without laughing nervously. Why? Because when we're doing a task, we're busy, but when we're asked to just "be," we feel uncomfortable—because we haven't been taught how to do that—yet.

As I said, there is never a time that a person with dementia can be wrong. Never. One time, I walked into a resident's room, and the person had stripped naked. Her room was turned upside down, and her clothes were strewn all over the place. The family was about to come in for a visit. And what did I say? I said, "Wow—this is great! Marge, look what you did! You changed the room around—I love it! I guess you didn't like what I had set out for you to wear—let's try this on." The object was not to make the person feel badly, because she was not doing this on purpose. That's one thing we tend to forget. These behaviors frustrate us, but believe me, if Marge could have changed back to how she was before the onset of the disease, she surely would have!

Look Inside Ourselves

We also need to remember that the only behavior we can change is our own. If a person had her cognitive abilities intact, she wouldn't have trashed her room, or gone into someone else's room and lay down in a strange bed, or grabbed food off someone else's tray. We need to remember that we're dealing with an illness that has inhabited a person, causing her to do these things.

A common question I'm asked: Does behavior modification work with someone who has dementia? The answer is: absolutely not! Think back to what we discussed earlier about the effects of dementia on an individual's brain. There's literally a hole created in the brain, and there's simply nothing there to replace what was once there—it's just gone. The brain has irrevocably lost its ability to carry out certain functions. That's why education and training have to constantly be reinforced among caregivers. Is it frustrating for the caregiver to have the person continually undo what they've just done? Sure it is, but we're not going to be able to reason this with this individual, and we can't expect him or her to change. If people with dementia could change, they surely wouldn't have this illness.

Chapter 9
Respecting an Individual's Personal Space

What's important for us to remember is that for every action, there's going to be a reaction. If we are caregivers, we need to come to work in a positive frame of mind and totally focused on enriching the lives of the people we care for.

In order for us to do this, our body language has to be "open" and welcoming. We don't want to be standing over somebody and telling them what to do, because that's very intimidating. Think about what it's like to be in a wheelchair, always having to look up at a person who's towering over you. We need to crouch down to their level. We need to make eye contact in order to feel their needs and experience them. That's why we need to remember to not hastily grab someone but rather, offer our hand.

In the early stages of getting to know residents, it's important to tell them your name and then say, "And your name is?" This gives them an opportunity to speak their own name and for you to repeat it back to them. "Oh! What a lovely name you have, Alice." "My mother's name is Alice, too!" "Let's go for a walk, Alice." The sound of one's name is deeply rooted in long-term memory, so when residents hear us calling them by name, they feel comforted and connected. That's why it's so important that whenever we engage residents in conversation, we address them by name as often as possible.

We also need to remember to make sure that our voice is pleasant, our facial expression is positive, and that we're not getting into the residents' personal space too quickly. We all know what feels comfortable in terms of our own personal space. We need to remember that this isn't any different for an individual with dementia. We need to look at the reactions of our residents in terms of when they think we're invading their personal space—and look for ways we can adjust our behaviors accordingly.

If you manage a dementia care unit and want a real-life demonstration to bring this concept home to your staff, try the following exercise.

Training Exercise: How Close Is Too Close?

You start this exercise by instructing your staff to form two lines about 20 feet apart and facing each other. Let the staff in one line play the role of the caregiver, and have the staff in the other line assume the role of the resident. Now instruct the "caregivers" that they will advance toward the "residents." But before you do, give the residents these instructions: "Put your hand up in front of you when you feel that the caregiver has come into your personal space, and the caregiver has to stop at that point." You'll see that the caregivers will not be in a straight line when the exercise is done; everyone has their own sense of when their personal space is being invaded. In this simple way, your staff will come to realize how everyone has a different concept of where his or her personal space or boundaries are.

We have to remember that several factors come into play in terms of whom we let into our personal space. For some residents, there could be a male/female issue or a cultural or race factor. For others, it could be a height issue—they might be intimidated by someone who's very tall—or it could be a weight issue—they become afraid when someone who's very large approaches them. We have to take all of that into account when we enter someone's personal space.

Establishing a Connection

I always tell caregivers to start making a personal connection from outside a person's room. That way, from the resident's point of view, we're not just walking in and getting him or her out of bed. We first make the connection by calling their name as we enter their room, and then offer our hand to them. The resident then gets used to us being in their personal space. When we think about it, our tendency in our daily lives is not to be right in a person's face. But when we're bathing someone, or assisting in the bathroom, we have no choice: physically we're very close. We have to be. That's why it's so important that we develop a re-spect for the person's space and understand the individual's level of comfort with us. Just because we're comfortable with them doesn't mean the person likes us intruding in their space!

As I said before, as caregivers we need to think about what we're learning. Every connection we make can teach us something about ourselves every single day—if we're open to it and allow it to happen. When we have someone resisting care or testing us in certain respects, we're learning about how to be more patient. I like to think of it in these terms: We have an opportunity to grow, to develop, and to learn something. We can even share what we've learned with the resident: "Michael, today you taught me that I really need to slow it down, and I can't thank you enough." "Florence, I could tell that you were getting irritated with me today by your body language. You really helped me today and I want to thank you for that." When you look at an experience in a new light, doesn't it make you think about what you can do differently next time?

It also gives us the opportunity to add "value" to individuals with dementia. By that. I mean they are acknowledged as people who can still teach us, share with us, and contribute to the world all around us. Simply put, they have value!

Caregivers Help to Create a Welcoming Environment

Caregivers need to understand that they are part of the environment, and what they bring to the environment is what makes the unit special. When we're telling caregivers to leave their problems at home when they come to work, what we're really saying is that your mood and your behaviors—both verbal and non-verbal—are going to affect the residents. A person with dementia is going to be very sensitive to our body language, for example. If we're having a bad day—and we're grouchy or impatient—the resident will pick up on that negative tone and react accordingly.

In terms of consistency within long-term care facilities, I always feel that permanent assignments will help both the caregiver and the resident. When the caregiver has worked with the same person, they will have the person's history and experience from their day to day encounters and will be able to take the best approach. Simply by starting out the day in a positive way with a familiar routine can bring about a level of care best suited for the person in need. For example, If I have never worked with you before I may not know that you like your coffee first thing in the morning, before any care is given and definitely before you sit down for your breakfast! I may not know that reading a letter to you from your daughter will bring about a smile and have a positive effect on your mood, start the day off in the right way. Both the caregiver and the resident benefit from knowing how the person wants to be treated. The resident's day starts off in a positive light and the caregiver's day as well. These daily occurrences help the caregiver gain knowledge about who the person truly is, understand his or her long-time rituals and habits, and value the individual as a person. This is how trust starts, and it's important to remember that trust only happens over time.

Chapter 10
Giving Purpose to the Way People Spend their Day

One of the obstacles we face in putting meaning into every-day living is a simple thing called a "calendar." Calendars dictate what we're going to do for the day. In long-term care facilities, a calendar fosters the mindset that we have to have prescribed arts and entertainment programs at certain times on certain days. (But in our everyday lives, do we plan out our leisure activities so rigorously? Absolutely not!) Granted, there are certain activities that can bring enjoyment—activities that can connect people and give people a purpose. But there is also something very thera-peutic about cleaning your house, or making your bed; doing the simple tasks of everyday life. But we don't see a great deal of that in terms of long-term care, where everything is done for the resi-dents.

The old way of thinking was, "we can't have people who live here do the work that we're supposed to be doing." Well, things have changed a lot since then! It can give people a sense of purpose simply to hang laundry outside on a clothesline, because when we put clothes on a line, think about all we do: we use our fingers to hang the clothes, watch with our eyes to make sure we've hung them correctly, and make small talk with others if there's more than one person doing the job. There's a sense of accomplish-ment created through doing the simplest of daily tasks. That's why giving a purpose to a resident's day is not all about organized activities that he or she may—or may not—want to participate in at a regimented time.

I see so many facilities spending thousands and thousands of dollars a year on scheduled activities instead of using that mon-ey differently. When I work with the administrators and staff of health care facilities, I always ask: "What would happen if you didn't have to use a calendar?" I'm not denying the fact that states require us to engage residents in certain activities. But instead of just having regular group activities, I advocate having what I call "discovery stations." These are areas around a unit where a nursing assistant could bring a resident so they could engage in an activity together. Some examples could be reading, painting, listening to music, looking at photos or art work, working with Fractiles®, or enjoying bird watching together. It could be a comfortable chair in the corner where they could just sit down together for a few minutes. These activities could be shared by any caregiver, team member, family member or volunteer wanting to spend time with the person.

Staff Example: Rob

Here's an example: Rob from Maintenance walks into the unit to fix a broken cabinet. He passes Ruth, who sits by a beautiful painting, gazing at it. He takes a moment to stop, looks at the painting and asks her questions about the colors that she likes. That's all it takes to have a meaningful interaction.

I've seen facilities where they have posted a set of questions in a hallway so anyone can start a conversation. In many facilities hallways are no longer just drab passageways filled with pictures nobody notices. Instead, hallways have become true discovery stations for display of artworks or interactive places for expression with purpose and intent. It's not just a hallway filled with pictures no one even notices—it's a true discovery station.

Discovery stations also present the perfect opportunity for us to develop opportunities that take residents outside into the fresh air. What if we were to structure a safe place—perhaps a landscaped garden with lush greenery, fragrant flowers, bird-feeders, and a gingerbread gazebo—where residents could stroll leisurely or sit comfortably in a tranquil natural setting. If people feel the need to walk, then let them have supervised experiences outside where they can experience nature—whether it's watching a chickadee at a bird feeder or a Monarch fluttering around a butterfly bush. It's a way for them to interact with the beauty nature offers all around us. We can get so caught up in our daily routines that we neglect to see beauty around us; let's not deprive them of the same experience. And best of all, these opportunities are free!

Personal Example: Janet

One resident I knew, Janet, always had a house filled with animals throughout her life. She needed the closeness and tenderness only a pet can give. The facility where she lived had a therapy dog named Sammy that gave Janet a sense of purpose in life. Grooming Sammy became part of her daily routine. One of the members of the housekeeping staff, who actually owned the dog, went through the requisite training to certify Sammy as a therapy dog. She would bring Sammy in every morning, and Janet's face would just light up. "He needs your love and brushing," Janet was told. With a huge smile, she immediately took to the task. Sammy not only added value to her day, but he gave her a purpose in life.

This type of practice is not hard to do, but it has to be taught and accepted as being part of the culture. There are many different ways to receive unconditional love and affection; pet therapy is a practice most of us are familiar with. But there are many others. Recently, I came across a robotic, animated seal named Paro that was developed by a Japanese industrial automation company called AIST.[13] The difference here is that the robotic seal allows individuals who have allergies, or a fear of cats or dogs, to enjoy the pleasure of tactile stimulation. I saw firsthand what it did for a woman who had great difficulty expressing herself verbally. When the soft, furry Paro was placed in her lap, she began to use words that were clear, audible and appropriate. As I said earlier, technology brings change to the healthcare field; this is a bona fide example of an advancement that has the potential to improve people's lives through touch, sound and movement.

Personal Example: Frank

It's easy to forget that people with dementia had a purpose in life prior to taking up residence at the facility. For example, I heard a story about an elderly man, Frank, who used to "make the rounds" of his floor every day, taking things from various people's rooms and depositing them at the nurse's station. (Frank was labeled "the taker.") After several attempts to get him to stop this behavior failed, the nurse looked through his initial admission form and found out that he had worked as a letter carrier for most of his adult life. The staff put their heads together and came up with an innovative idea: they created a makeshift delivery route for Frank, complete with envelopes laid out each morning at various "stops" and a basket at the nurse's station for him to make his "deliveries" every afternoon. Sometimes he delivered the daily activity schedule; other times it was a poem, the newspaper or the daily menu. This type of approach stopped people's things from disappearing, and gave Frank a purpose in life again.

Personal Example: Betty

Betty was a new resident in the dementia unit who was very frustrated and angry upon her arrival. She would pace the halls for hours and did not want to engage in any of the planned recreational activities. Because her family had provided the facility with a thorough background history, we found out that Betty had 10 children. As one of her children said, Betty was always standing by the sink, one hand on the faucet washing dishes with the other rocking a baby to and fro. We talked about Betty's history with the staff, and one nursing assistant hesitantly suggested we set up a small nursery in the building with a crib, bassinet and dolls. I say "hesitantly," because the nursing assistant thought her idea might be too childlike, since we were providing elder care. Well, we had a feeling this might be just what Betty needed, and sure enough, it was. You could see it in Betty's face as soon as she was handed a doll to cradle in her arms. A smile came over her face and she relaxed—she was in her glory, back in a time when she felt safe and secure. Thanks to that nursing assistant's idea, Betty now felt at home.

Personal Example: Dr. Jeffrey

There's one last story I want to share here about "Dr. Jeffrey." He was a resident at a facility where the staff knew of his background as a therapist. They would come up to him and say things like, "Dr Jeffrey, I wanted to share my issues with you today and see if you could help." Although he could no longer speak, you could see in his eyes that he was listening. At the end of the conversation, the staff member would reach for his hands and say, "Thank you, sharing this with you helped me." One day a staff member noticed both a tear and a smile on his face.

Clearly, if we're open to them, there are numerous opportunities available each day to enrich the lives of people with dementia.

Creating More Opportunities to Interact

At long-term care facilities, there needs to be a way of interacting on the dementia unit, without always having a scheduled activity, so the entire team can get to know each other in meaningful ways. This will better enable staff at these facilities to enrich the lives of the residents. Let me describe what I mean: If I'm a nurse, and my primary role is to give you medication, I'll walk over to you with the intent of administering the meds. I'll check to see that you are right person, tell you it's your medication time and give you your pills. But if my intention is to first communicate with you and make a connection, my action would be something like this: I start our conversation with a good morning, letting you know my name, and asking what you would like to be called. I give you a sincere compliment, spend a moment talking with you and then proceed to give your medication. Do you see the difference?

The same practice needs to take place with all the members on the team. Take the housekeeper whose job is to clean the room, for example. She could be taught to first say hello, connect with the resident and spend a few minutes talking with him or her before cleaning their room. It could be about something as simple as a picture on the wall or knickknack on a shelf. Is this a different role? Actually, yes it is. It takes a person's job beyond being just focused on the task. When this practice is fully integrated into the culture, everyone understands and accepts that the task and the connection hold equal importance.

I feel the nursing assistant's title should reflect the specialized training that needs to be part of this new role. A nursing assistant's role working with cognitive patients in a short-term rehab facility is much different than the role of the nursing assistant on a dementia unit—and it should be. As I have said before, if their training is specialized, and their care is specialized, then let's reflect that in their titles as well.

It reminds me of a time when primary nursing was the norm in the 1970s before we had a medication nurse and other nursing specialties. The nurse cared for the person in every way. The same holds true here. I'm not saying to do away with positions like recreation therapists; what I am saying is that we need to orient our staff differently. One recreation therapist cannot be the only person in charge of a person's well being or social needs! That's why a team approach is needed to enable the cross-training of staff. We need to teach the nursing assistants, as well as everyone else on the Dementia Care team, to make every engagement a meaningful one. These types of added responsibilities need to be built into the job descriptions to reflect the new culture.

The following is a wonderful example of what I'm talking about.

Staff Example: Stacey

Stacey, a nursing assistant, knew that one particular resident's favorite song was "Over the Rainbow." Stacey would come into the room with a smile on her face, nothing in her hands, and say "good morning" to the resident. Stacey proceeded to look into the resident's eyes with a smile and sing "Over the Rainbow" to her. The resident, who was non-verbal, swayed back and forth to the music with a smile. Talk about a meaningful engagement! For those few moments the resident felt happy and connected.

Stacey then got a warm cloth and proceeded to wash the resident's face while still singing the song.

Often, we make plans for recreational activities and try to get the residents to participate. But if I were looking at where I'd want to spend some of my recreation budget, I would look at the needs of the residents first, and then base my programming around them.

In summary, if I am a nurse in charge of a unit and am responsible for 40 residents, I should know enough about each of them to understand what makes each one happy, just like Stacey, the nursing assistant in my last example, did. I should know that getting outside every day makes Hank, a former grounds keeper, really happy. I should know that Mrs. Smith in Room 329 loves animals—in fact, she had pets her whole life. And I should know that the newest resident, Arthur, played the drums throughout his life, starting in the military right through to the senior citizens' center.

Chapter 11
Developing an Effective Team Through Cross-training

We've discussed the need to look for ways to change the mindset of having prescribed activities at prescribed times. Here's why: Often, residents in long-term care facilities will experience what we call "sun-downing." Late in the afternoon, they tend to get nervous because they're bored, restless, and/or simply tired. The residents may not know where they're supposed to be going or what they're supposed to be doing. The shifts are changing; there's a lull before dinner while all new staff are coming in for the evening. The recreation therapist is typically going home for the day. There is activity, but the residents aren't necessarily a part of it.

These are the times that we need to make sure things are taking place to engage the residents as well. We need to implement creative solutions that involve cross-training the staff in new and unique ways.

The recreation therapist's role is to engage residents so they have things to do. If this is the case, then I contend that the recreation therapist needs to be working with Nursing in a different way. In some facilities, Recreation and Nursing team up to collaborate on the day's events and plan programs. Recreation staff may lead the team, but with the support of all team members from various departments. The team leader needs to be trained properly to perform this role. For example, some residents may enjoy sleeping late, while others may be early risers. Can the two groups be accommodated?

Leading a True "Team"

To be considered a team, we have to work together tightly as a unit, seeing the big picture and not just the task at hand. It requires cross training, for sure—if you want to have a specialized unit, then you have to have staff well-versed in many different skills.

Teaching a team leader to break down barriers of what's considered a nursing job and what's considered a recreation therapist's job requires redefining roles if we're to truly change the culture. For example, nursing assistants need to be taught about how to use conversational starters, engage a person, and find common bonds. The same goes for Housekeeping, Laundry, Dietary and Maintenance. While it may sound like common sense, all of these groups must learn how to do this. Learning these new skills takes time and effort.

I recently observed a class that one of my close friends conducted with residents of a dementia unit. I was amazed at how she phrased her questions and the way she introduced a topic. The residents looked at pictures from their eras, and she engaged each one with the right word, the right touch and the right look. She was able to get everyone involved even if some didn't have verbal skills anymore. The way she did this—her performance—was truly inspirational. I learned so much from my friend just by watching how effortlessly she engaged the residents in so many different ways and by observing how skillfully she had accomplished this goal. I felt equally inspired when I noticed a nursing assistant artfully move a patient with great ease, because I know how difficult it is to position someone without pushing and pulling. Both my friend and the nursing assistant had taken the time necessary to develop their exceptional caregiving talents, but because they took that time, they now have impressive skill sets to work with.

Because of the traditional separation of roles and duties associated with nursing assistants, we don't get to see the full spectrum of what staff members are capable of accomplishing. Conversely, when they solely focus day in and day out on such tasks as bathing, feeding, toileting and dressing, nursing assistants aren't able to see the residents' other capabilities. What they're seeing with their concentration on basic tasks is only one dimension of the person—not the whole person. The same goes for the recreation assistant, who may not be aware of the resident's personal care habits and routines. It's important to remember that each team member's unique strengths and expertise are what makes a facility truly unique. We need to look for ways to capitalize on these strengths in order to improve the resident's quality of life.

Overlapping Roles and Responsibilities

We need to think about overlapping roles and responsibilities of our staff, wherever possible, to benefit the individuals under our care. For example, if a buffet breakfast was offered and served by all team members—such as dietary, nurses, housekeeping and recreation staff—could it lead to a more leisurely-paced dining experience? Think about it: Breakfast could become a time for socializing, perhaps by discussing current events or just listening to great music. Couldn't we try this type of approach instead of rushing to get everyone to a formal recreation program? By looking at overlapping shift routines for the Recreation Department, could we better accommodate residents' needs? Could we provide more activities in the late afternoon and after meal time? And if a quiet evening program were initiated, would it encourage better sleep?

Think about it: The recreation therapist would be more effective working with the nursing staff, even on a limited basis, to show them how to engage the residents on a more routine basis. The certified nursing assistant—familiar with the person's habits and patterns—would ensure that the recreation program or activity is at a time best suited for the resident. The CNA would continue to ensure that the resident is washed, dressed and ready for when the recreation therapist takes over.

We have to be sure that we all are part of creating an environment that supports the person. If someone is sitting in a chair with nothing to do, and you know he or she likes flowers, then have a book with garden photos close by so that as a care partner, you can share the experience. It can be that simple.

Personal Example: Lilly

Lilly was a 78-year-old former elementary school teacher who was always looking for Bijou, the dog she had many years ago when she was younger. Recreation staff knew that Lilly loved spending time with the facility's therapy dog. They also knew that she loved singing along to her favorite song, "She'll Be Coming Around the Mountain." Both activities put Lilly in a great mood.

But the nursing staff didn't know about this. What they did know, however, was that it was a daily struggle to get Lilly dressed in time for the recreation program — which, ironically, was music and singing. One day a nursing assistant was talking to one of the recreation assistants and found out about Lilly's favorite song and her love for dogs. With this new knowledge about what cheered up Lilly, the nursing assistant took it upon herself to sing "She'll Be Coming Round the Mountain" to Lilly while getting her dressed. A broad smile came across Lilly's face. That same assistant then sought out the facility dog and brought it to see Lilly regularly. Once the nursing assistant knew these vital pieces of information, because she'd spoken to the recreation assistant and responded accordingly, Lilly's quality of life dramatically improved.

Start With One Resident at a Time

Think about what it would be like if you created a care plan ensuring a fulfilling day for one resident based on what you knew about him or her. Think about how you would schedule your time if you had that freedom.

Now look at some tiny steps you can take to make someone's day more fulfilling. Many different jobs and tasks can be incorporated into the daily routines of our residents. Simple assignments, such as setting tables or folding table linens and towels, can give someone a sense of purpose. The same goes for filling baskets with flowers for table arrangements during meal times.

If somebody loves to talk, then let that person be the greeter for people coming into the dining room. Even helping with clean up can make someone feel useful and needed. We all need to have a purpose in life, and in that "all," please remember to include individuals with dementia—we can't forget that they, too, need to have purpose. That's why we must start looking at each department in a different light and then find ways that residents can be involved in the process. This can only be done by working together, not in isolation.

Schedules are typically based on 8 a.m. to 5 p.m. or 9 a.m. to 5 p.m. shifts in Recreation, OT, PT or office jobs. I don't see very many evening or weekend programs in dementia care units because the staff works day shifts, with weekends off. Again, as caregivers, what are we here for? But I was pleased when I saw one program offering "night daycare" for people who have always been night owls. Instead of using sleep medication to get residents' schedules to conform to our ways, the staff rearranged their schedules to work with the residents' schedules. This exemplifies an effort to meet the residents' true needs and to enable a better way of life.

I'm sure people will read this and ask, "How can you accommodate everyone?" The simple answer is that you can't, of course— but this one program's way of thinking should make the rest of us stop and look at our current schedules. Think about it: Can we stagger shifts? Can we have a program before bed that would help to promote sleep? Can we offer massages for the back, feet and hands? Can quiet music be part of a bedtime program? I can hear you say, "Who has the time?" Well, if with intention we are working in a different way—with respectful and caring practices— then we will have a lot more time freed up. We won't be writing as many incident reports, taking as many people to the hospitals or distributing extra medications for unwanted behaviors. We need to reward the staff who make the effort to enrich the residents' lives and not just rush to complete their duties by a certain time. Simply put, we need to acknowledge staff for care well done, with intention. This is part of changing the culture.

At this point, I feel it's important to point out that I'm not advocating a huge staff or resource expansion to enable this true culture change to happen. Long-term care facilities need to focus on their current resources—not on what they don't have. People always say, "If only we had more staff we could do this so much better..." Well, I feel differently!

One way you can take stock of the resources you already have is by stepping outside your front door.

A New Culture Is in the Air

I'd like you to think about what it would be like not to get out of your house for days at a time. You wouldn't smell the fresh air, feel the wind, or hear the leaves rustling. Think about how you feel when you're closed in for an extended period of time.

When I lecture, I'm typically in a building most of the day for three days at a time. How does that make me feel? Confined. Oxygen-deprived. Sometimes, I even feel claustrophobic. Now think about a resident of a dementia care unit. As part of my work, I regularly see areas outside physical buildings where residents who are ambulatory can sit. But people in dementia units rarely get out much. In fact, people in late stage dementia don't get out at all. Yet we all need to get some fresh air, even if it's only for a few minutes at a time. This understanding needs to be part of our new culture.

I'd like to pose this question: How often do we have picnics outside—or even breakfast or snacks—in the warm summer months or in the cool autumn air? How often do our physical therapists take our residents outside and have their programs there? (If not, why not?) If inmates in state prisons are mandated to have at least one hour of outside recreation per day, why aren't people in long-term care afforded the same privilege? Just because someone can't walk, why should they be deprived of this enriching experience?

Instead of having someone come inside to lead an activity, I would much rather see volunteers—whether it's children, teenagers or people from the community—take the residents outside and use nature as a way to entertain them.

The Audubon Society has wonderful resources to help with these kinds of activities. It can be something as simple as talking about the trees and the seasons, feeling the air, walking or feeding the birds. It's all about having an interaction. You can give residents simple tasks, such as filling bird feeders and planting flowers. Even in the winter you can have residents take on that role inside by watering plants. I advocate providing a live plant for each resident in a facility. The plant is there to be nurtured, enjoyed and shared with others. In return, it gives the resident a sense of purpose, so he or she can wake up in the morning and have something to look after. (Yes, even for people with dementia.) It's something they can share with others and together enjoy its beauty.

As caregivers, we all need to think about this: What would it be like for us to wake up tomorrow morning and be confined to a chair? What would we do all day long? How many people would come to see us? Would we feel isolated? We might have one certified nursing assistant who would be the only person we'd see that whole day. And if we didn't like her, we wouldn't be very happy, would we?

Expand the 'World' for Someone with Dementia

As I've mentioned, the world for people with dementia shrinks as the disease progresses. Their verbal skills decrease and their ability to initiate conversations and personal interactions dwindles. What if we set out intentionally to expand their immediate world by adding people who know something about them? If each staff member who entered the unit stopped and said hello to a resident for a few minutes each day, that person's world would grow, become more interesting and include more positive, meaningful interactions. Like I said, this does not entail adding staff—it entails expanding the role each person plays in enriching the resident's quality of life.

Think of the people who come on the unit each day—the housekeeper, the recreation therapist, the physical therapist, the dietician, the secretary, the volunteer, the family member -- do you see where I am going? You've already got a multi-faceted team in place at a typical long-term care facility. People from diverse backgrounds are people with great ideas and diverse points of view. Pairing each resident up with one or two people from this interdisciplinary team will extend that person's social network, so they're not just seeing their nursing assistant over the course of a day. They may be seeing Jennifer, the dietary manager who loves dogs. Or Harold, the maintenance man who has the heartiest laugh and gives the most wonderful hugs—he is also quite handsome. And as he compliments the women on the unit, they smile from ear to ear!

A facility that's going to be successful with this approach needs to have every staff member be a team member. Why? When you're truly changing a culture, people find out who their colleagues and customers really are. I advise facilities to start by having their staff get to know each other, as I've mentioned earlier. Once this happens and they've had some practice, it's time to apply this approach with the residents. I see it as more than just a way to establish a common bond—it's a way for us all to relate on a more human level, person to person.

The Effects of Positive Interactions

If the positive effects of these interactions I've mentioned still aren't enough to convince you that a change is needed, think about this: Research published in the April 2010 journal PNAS, Proceedings of the National Academy of Sciences, found that the emotion tied to a memory lingers in the mind even after the memory is gone.(14) Justin Feinstein, a graduate student in neuropsychology at the University of Iowa, conducted an experiment where he threw a movie festival at the hospital where he works. Feinstein chose clips from tear-jerkers such as "Forrest Gump." After the movie, the patients did not remember seeing the movie, but still they felt sad. Feinstein repeated the experiment but this time, instead of using sad moments, he played cheerful and uplifting clips. Sure enough—when the movie was over, the patients didn't remember a thing about it, but their general mood was upbeat. Emotions outlasted the memories once again.

Individuals with dementia may not remember why they feel good after having a positive interaction with others, but they'll know that positive emotional response came from somewhere— and just knowing that instinctively can be enough to provide comfort for someone with dementia.

Chapter 12
Making a Home Feel Like Home

We've discussed several concepts relating to culture change that involve looking at people and processes in a new light. Now that we've laid some of the groundwork for change, we need to think about how we can provide a culture that embraces home in the purest and simplest form. For people who will not be going back to their own homes, how can we make their new surroundings feel like home?

When we think about home, we think about a place where we can wear sloppy clothes and not comb our hair if we don't want to. I recall an old saying that describes this feeling perfectly: "Home is the place where it feels right to walk around without shoes." That's because we relax at home—it's the place that provides us with comfort.

We need to remember that feeling when we're working with people who have dementia. If these individuals' rooms are to now be considered their "home," then their personal space needs to reflect that. Their rooms should not feel like they're in an institution. Instead, their rooms should be places where they can feel at home and be comfortable, even if they don't want to be around other people.

What are the essentials? A chair, comforter, sheets and pillow that provide a sense of comfort are needed, for starters. We all like to have comfortable things around us that make us feel good, and every person—with or without dementia—deserves the best. If you're living in a long-term care facility, it's likely to be the last place you're going to live. As caregivers, we need to ensure that we have comfort measures in place for these individuals, whether families can provide for them or not. Each room needs to signify the comfort of the individual's own home.

When we walk into someone's home, we automatically get a sense of what the person is like through their style of furniture, color schemes, plants and family photos, to name a few. What does their home say about them? The same feeling should come through when we walk into someone's room, or shared space. Think about what's hung on the walls—are there pictures of things this person likes, are the colors ones that the person living there would pick out?

Many times in older buildings you'll have two people sharing a room. This may be a very small space, but we can still make the most of the surroundings and personalize them. This is where having an in-depth history is important; it enables us to make the room feel individualized, even if it's half of a room.

Personal Example: Rose

Recently I met Rose, who was a painter. She had been admitted into a long-term care facility, and her room had scenes of water and boats all around her. Walking into her room, I immediately thought she must have lived near the water, or maybe enjoyed boating. But what I found out was that Rose had a near death experience as a teenager and almost drowned. The pictures were in the room before she moved in, and no one had looked at them to question if they would be the right fit.

The truth was, Rose was afraid of the water, so when caregivers walked into her room and started a conversation about the beach and water scenes, Rose would become upset and start to yell. It wasn't until we spoke to the family that we found out Rose had had a bad experience in her youth.

This proves once again why asking the right questions and having an in-depth history is so critical to our care. Personalizing the space is something that goes hand in hand with person-centered care. We should have things on the wall that reflect what the person appreciates. Think about our living room or bedroom, for example. What provides us with comfort? What do we enjoy looking at? We should put the same thought into decorating the rooms for people we care for.

Honoring One's Space

We need to remember that when we're in an individual's room, we need to honor his or her space. This is not our time to turn the radio to a station we like or turn the television volume down. It's about respecting personal space and knowing what a person needs in that small area to make it feel like home.

Some of us who work in health care facilities don't even realize that we're dishonoring a person's home when we're doing it. There might be trash cans cluttering the floor and plastic institutional pitchers and basins taking up space. Can't we remove some of these institutional obstacles and replace them with more personal things? Or, is there a storage bench or a closed shelf where some of these items could be stored out of the way and out of sight until they're needed?

It could even be as simple as getting rid of the plastic mugs that serve drinks at meal time. Why not serve coffee and tea in real china? It certainly would feel more homelike to me. In the past, we looked for mugs that would maintain the temperature of hot beverages since meals were delivered on trays. Today, facilities are employing more of a home style dining approach, with coffee poured at the table. This is the perfect time to serve residents in their favorite china mugs or teacups. I know I have a favorite mug I use—why can't they?

I remember one nursing assistant who was great at making things tidy. Any room she worked in had a certain order and function. She could make an untidy room look immaculate by getting rid of clutter, which we're told is a good thing to do for small places. She worked with one resident who enjoyed having photos on the bedside table of her children. She also loved fresh flowers there, as well as her tissue box. But to this caregiver, that was pure clutter! This is why we need to once again remember what we're doing, why we're doing it, and how our actions must have meaning for the person in our care. It's all about what makes a room actually feel like someone's "home." And we have to remember that to some people, their clutter makes them feel comfortable and at home.

A Unique Vantage Point

I always ask staff at various facilities I work with to go into a resident's room, lie down on the bed, and assess the arrangement of the room from this vantage point. One of my memories from childhood is my mother doing this in our guest room before overnight visitors arrived. It was—and still is—a good way to make sure someone has all necessities within easy reach in order to be comfortable..

The more that we simplify one's surroundings and remove institutional staples, the less institutional a person's room will feel. Sometimes a number of our institutional furnishings aren't even needed, but we don't question them—they're a given. For example, what is the bedside table used for? Do we really need it? A resident can't even reach it when lying on the bed. If we could begin to question things like this, it's a start. Isn't there a more functional side table that could suit the same purpose? If a person wants to sit in a chair and have a meal alone, can't we make the room more suitable for this instead of using an institutional tray stand? There are many types of small, round tables that would be perfect for this.

Outside organizations are happy to create handmade goods, such as crocheted lap blankets, to make residents' rooms more personalized. If residents don't have family, then we need to take it upon ourselves to find things to make their rooms more homey. This reflects a facility that really does care by replacing an institutional focus with an intentional focus on the individual.

The following categories reflect several environmental dimensions that we need to pay careful attention to in order to create truly comfortable surroundings.

Music and Photos

Music is a lifeline for people with dementia, as they can feel the music. It soothes them and brings back memories, establishing a time and place. But the music has to be personal, so it's important to develop individualized music histories for people with dementia. The University of Iowa has done some pioneering work with music assessments, finding that individualized music can significantly alleviate agitation in individuals with dementia.

We have to make sure the music we're using as a form of therapy and enjoyment is music the person likes. Otherwise, it can make them extremely uncomfortable.

In every stage of this disease—whether it's early, middle or late—people lose more of their functioning ability. It's critical to ensure that we continue to stimulate them with such things as music so they can still connect with and find a sense of meaning.

Most of us are comfortable when we have things around us that are familiar. That's why people with dementia also need to have personal things around them to make them feel safer. The more we can personalize their area, the more secure they will be. Things that tell a story—photos, for example—are important. I encourage family members to put together inexpensive photo albums that residents can carry in their pockets. Family photos can be a great conversation starter, allowing us to engage them both verbally and non-verbally by pointing to the people pictured. So can memory boxes and even digital frames with constantly changing photos.

Using family photographs and music are just two ways to offer residents reassurance and support, which is so important in every single stage of this illness. There is no time when these individuals should be left without stimulation, no matter what stage of the illness they're experiencing. It's important to remember they can still show us something about themselves, about caregiving, about relationships and about love until the very end.

Sound

When we're working in long term care facilities, it's not uncommon to see a group of residents just sitting there—most of the time outside the nurse's station—not listening to music, not watching TV, not looking outside. They've got the overhead pagers blaring in their ears. Workers are whizzing by, performing their daily routines. When you see something like this happening, stop and think about how uncomfortable these people must be. Might they be better off their own room, with some soft music on and feet propped up under a warm blanket, looking out the window? If somebody loves music, but the music bothers a roommate, there are alternatives. You can make sure all music lovers have comfortable headsets for listening to their favorite music, which will provide a calming effect. Regularly check the volume level of your residents music playing devices and make sure batteries are in good working order. There are even pillows that have been designed with a speaker inside to make it more comfortable to hear music, such as the Sound Oasis® sleep therapy pillow. Again, it's up to us to be creative in these types of situations.

Another source of sound—in this case, noise—emanates from the nurse's station. And it's not a soothing sound! I feel strongly that there's no reason to have a nurse's station on every floor. Nursing stations often create a barrier that gives the impression it's "we" versus "them." Residents in wheelchairs can't even see the person behind the desk, and to my mind, the only purpose this station serves is for charting. Today, with all the technological advances that have been made—as evidenced by portable phones, computerized charting, and medicine cabinets in everyone's rooms—we can re-design this space as living space for residents.

We have to remember to ask ourselves: whose home is this, anyway? I've seen several older buildings—and modern buildings where physical changes can't be made right away—where creative ways have been found to modify the space formerly occupied by a nursing station. I've seen this space used as an art center for painting simply by lowering the counter's height so it is level with the desk portion. When this is done, the space can be used for arts and crafts and letter writing, to name but a few. Another facility used this space to set up a store for people who like to shop. They added different shelves and racks to store clothes, drawers to rummage through and organize, and flat surfaces on which to fold laundry. I've also seen these spaces converted into mini-museums, with artwork hanging on the outside and shelves to hold flowers, books and other things to look at.

There are many creative ways to redesign a space. If you eliminate the nurse's station, it can become the perfect space for residents to come together. If we set it up and adapt it well, properly placing furniture and lighting, then these areas can serve as small, intimate spaces that would invite conversation and relaxation. You don't need to go out and buy new furniture to do this; use what you have. Find something that resembles a coffee table to serve as the focal point and spread books and magazines out on it. Again, be creative!

Furniture Placement

When we talk about the placement of the furniture, it's critical to make sure it's done in the most conducive manner to make the resident feel comfortable. In her book "Notes on Nursing," Florence Nightingale wrote about how a nurse's role is to ensure that every angle and every aspect of a person's room should facilitate healing and make the resident feel loved and respected.

If you have an ability to put the bed facing out a window, for example, then this is the perfect way to bring nature into one's surroundings. It's a beautiful way to live in concert with nature. Do we even think about this when we arrange a person's room? Most of the time, we don't even think about the placement of furniture—it's a static setup. Sometimes you can't even move the bed because of the way the room is situated with the headboard mounted to the wall or lighting that is stationary overhead. But is the sitting chair mounted to the wall? No! So move that chair around so the person can look out the window—simple as that. Creativity is defined as looking at the same thing everyone else sees but thinking something different. Be the person who sees beyond the institution.

The Bathroom

It's just as important to remember that the individual's bathroom is considered their "space," just as his or her bedroom is, so try to make it as homey as possible. Buy a colored shower curtain; put some pictures up in the bathroom that the person would like. Do your homework: use the resident background files to determine their interests. Use that knowledge to buy some wall art that reminds them of something familiar. We need to be sure to place items of interest at eye level. If you're not sure, sit in a wheelchair and see what it would look like from the resident's viewpoint. Have towels that are fluffy and colored instead of those white institutional towels that are rough on your skin and uninviting. Provide a warm bathrobe and terry wraps. Many times families want to bring in gifts but don't know what to buy. Give them ideas! How about a portable towel warmer? Or a soft, plush lap blanket? Other functional product resources can be found through Brookstone (*See Additional Resources,* **Websites**).

Lighting

It's important to think about the lighting in an individual's room—both the source, and the direction it's coming from. Often, fluorescent lights are located on the wall where the headboard is located, above the person's head. That's simply the worst kind of lighting. You need directional light for someone with dementia to see what they're reading or holding in their hand. It's difficult for us to comprehend what a person with a visual impairment actually sees. When you couple a condition like glaucoma with a disease like dementia, it makes it all the more complicated to see.

Caregivers need to be sensitive to how it feels to live with impaired vision. There is an excellent resource called Vision Simulations (*See Additional Resources*, **Websites**) that family members and caregivers can use to experience what it's like to live with a particular visual impairment. It's one way to walk a mile in the person's shoes, as I said at the beginning of the book, and get a sense of what a person truly "sees."

I always ask staff to go in the room of a visually impaired resident and think about what features of the room might need to be changed or adjusted in order to enhance the occupant's quality of life. Sometimes a simple shift in the direction of the light may make all the difference in what a person can or cannot see.

Personal Example: Virginia

I recall walking into the room of a resident who had just moved into an assisted living facility. Family members had put a lot of thought into the move; they brought many personal mementos, family photos and furniture from home. But what did they forget? Lamps! Virginia loved to read and do word search puzzles to pass the time, but could only do so during daylight hours because her chair was positioned near the window. However, Virginia hardly ever had time to sit by the window and read during the day, since most of her daytime hours were filled with planned activities outside the room. In the evening, when she finally had time to sit down and read a book or complete a puzzle, the small globe light outside her bathroom door provided very poor illumination. Problem solved: a simple trip to a home improvement store procured a standing floor lamp and a 27" tall table lamp, complete with three-way bulbs so the lighting could be adjusted. When the new lamps were plugged-in, a warm glow flooded the room, and a happy Virginia settled into her recliner with her puzzle book and proclaimed, "Now this feels like home!"

Colors and Contrasts

One thing we know is that color contrasting is also very important for people with dementia. They suffer occipital lobe damage, which, as I mentioned before, affects their vision. A good rule to follow here is to be sure to highlight—in a contrasting color—the thing you want to be noticed. Visual impairments are known to cause confusion and stress. When "colors" are simply white on white, for example, they form a single dimension for a person with dementia. Think about how this applies to a person's bathroom, for example. Imagine being in a bathtub. The attending nursing assistant is wearing a uniform with a white scrub top that blends into the surroundings. You're trying to find the white soap on a white soap dish against white tile. Now if there were a color contrast—the soap dish was blue with a bar of white soap on it, for example—you'd be able to see the soap and find it much faster.

What else do you have inside a typical long-term care facility? You've got white toilets, white sinks and white linens—just about everything is white! We've always been taught that white is good—it's clean and sanitary. But if someone with dementia is looking for a toilet and it's white and blends in with the surroundings, then they're going to have a hard time. That's why it's important to remove or replace white objects with brightly colored ones as much as possible. Paint the wall a bright color. Install brightly colored toilet seats. Make that contrast visible! I recall one resident who always used to urinate in a large green planter outside of his room. Why? Because he could see it! The toilet simply was not visible to him until we painted the wall red, and then the white seat stood out!

Another thing to be careful of is anything with a pattern: if the person has a visual impairment or is experiencing delirium, they might think tiny polka dots are bugs moving around. If we want to employ a pattern, we need to think about what it could look like to a person with dementia. A very easy rule to think about is that when babies are born, the only thing their eyes can detect are large contrasts between light and dark or black and white. It's the same for people with dementia, although they can see contrasting colors as well.

A Familiar Presence

When you've done everything you can to make the room as comfortable and homey as possible, there's another thing to remember: you can still find ways to tap into a person's long-term memory. Many times a way to accomplish this is by going back to a familiar song or a familiar voice that will bring out a positive emotional response.

For example, people tend to calm down when they hear the reassuring voice of a family member. A way to accomplish on an "as needed" basis is to create a DVD, make a talking scrapbook (I've seen these in retail stores) or record your voice on a talking photograph frame. The latter two products are readily available on line. The DVD will take a little more work on your part, but will be even more reassuring. I've even come across companies that put together digital life stories such as Reflection Connection (*See Additional Resources*, **Websites**).

It's common today for many families to have camcorders. If you want to create a lasting memory to reassure your loved one when you're not there, here's what you can do: set up the camera on a tripod, hit the record button and talk into the camera, addressing the person by name. As I said earlier, people with dementia often remember their name until the very end. Whether it's hearing your voice—or seeing you on a TV screen—it will be more comforting for the individual than you can possibly know. What's even better is to capture several members of your family on video, talking to the person. DVD players are quite common today in these types of facilities; it's possible to have one connected to the TV by the person's bedside. When someone's having a hard day, it's a great device for the caregiver to use to calm the person down. What better way to feel comfortable and at home than to see and hear familiar voices of those you hold dear?

It also gives the caregiver the perspective of seeing that this person had a wonderful life—and that's something staff members seldom see.

Chapter 13
An Overlooked Pathway—Dining

*"Sharing food with another human being is an intimate act
that should not be indulged in lightly."*

M.F.K. Fisher

I firmly believe that perhaps the most important quality of a dementia unit is its dining program. Food is the essence of life. Sharing food is an essential part of every culture—a part of civilization as we know it—and an important part of life. Meal times represent important rituals in everyone's life. In relation to our quality of life, dining is a major part of how we spend our day and plays a significant role in making us feel at home in our surroundings.

But all too often, dining is viewed in institutional settings as a form of medicine. What do I mean by that? The focus is placed on calories, vitamins and the amount of food someone consumes. But a meal is more than simply consuming calories and nutrients—it's an ideal time to establish a common bond between the caregiver and the resident.

This requires both a change in the process and a change in the way things have always been done. Why? Simply put, because dining needs to be viewed as a time for socialization and companionship. It's one of the most important activities of the entire day and one of the key elements necessary for true culture change.

When you or I sit down to a meal with our family or friends, what's the first thing we do? Do we simply eat what's on our plate? Is our mind set on getting the food into our bodies and nothing else? Likely not! Let's face it: breakfast, lunch and dinner are part of our daily rituals. As a result, there are certain aspects that we've come to enjoy: food that tastes good and is appealing, conversation that is easy and free-flowing, and surroundings that make meal times something we look forward to.

We know that every time we eat, it's not always in an ideal setting—we lead busy lives; we're often rushing to get to our next appointment or activity. But think about the last time you ate something you hated, just to eat. Or the last time you sat with someone with whom you had nothing in common, or felt no connection with, through an entire meal. Or the last time you ate in a restaurant where the surroundings were jarring, the noise was too loud, or worse, the environment begged you to hurry up and get out.

Dining: A Time to Bond

If you're like me, the scenarios I mentioned typically aren't the norm. In virtually every culture, meal time is shared with family and friends, which establishes a common bond that becomes part of our daily routines.

Now think about individuals with dementia. If they're in an institutional setting, they're likely not living with family or life-long friends. That's why it's critical to re-create that common bond they experienced earlier in their lives—before the onset of dementia—to make food as much a source of emotional nourishment as it is physical nourishment.

"Dining with Grace"

A few years ago I developed a program called "Dining with Grace" that revolves around dining with a spirit that fosters beauty, kindness and honor. It recognizes that dining offers physical, emotional, spiritual and sensory experiences.

Many times, people with dementia are not able to begin the meal because they have lost the ability to start eating. Caregivers often take this as a sign that they need to assist the resident, taking away one more piece of their independence. Before we do this, we need to ask ourselves some important questions: Can they see the silverware? Is the place setting in their range of vision? Are there too many utensils, causing confusion? Can they still hold a utensil? If the caregiver simply guides the movement of putting a fork or spoon to one's mouth, many times the person will continue themselves, with intermittent cueing. Also, a person may keep his or her independence longer if served creative types of finger foods.

We also need to ask ourselves if there is sufficient contrast so a person with dementia can actually see his or her food. Just think about the way a table is usually set—white table linens, white napkins and white dishes. And often, what color is the food that goes on those dishes? Mashed potatoes . . . cauliflower . . . chicken . . . vanilla ice cream.

It is important that we examine what's happening during mealtime; as a person's skills deteriorate, more and more of his or her actions will be performed by someone else. But we want an individual to remain independent for as long as possible throughout the course of this illness. That's why meals simply shouldn't be rushed, and that's why we must change the length of meal times to encourage independence and create an environment that fosters communication, companionship and sharing.

Eating a meal while someone is staring at you—and not partaking in the experience—is uncomfortable. We all have experienced residents who want you to take a bite of food along with them. They're telling us something if we'll only listen—this is wisdom that they're providing. Staff members need to be encouraged to at least drink a beverage while the resident is eating.

Culture change is about changing the institutional model into one that's familiar. Dining needs to be viewed as a shared experience. This has not historically been the practice, but today, it's being practiced more and more—especially in smaller facilities.

Factors to Consider

We need to realize up front that meal time can present several challenges, with individuals doing one or more of the following:

- not staying in the dining room, instead wanting to get up and walk away
- appearing anxious and restless
- holding food in their mouth, forgetting to chew and or swallow
- grabbing food from other people's trays

Additionally, external environmental factors may make the experience less than appetizing. There may be loud, jarring announcements heard on the overhead paging system. In addition, nursing assistants may be talking to each other or raising their voices to get individuals to eat.

Individuals with dementia are typically grouped together by their need for assistance as opposed to their need for socialization. When was the last time you had to sit next to someone at a social gathering who you couldn't wait to get away from? Now imagine if that was your everyday ritual . . . would that entice you to eat, or do just opposite? Why should this scenario be any different among individuals with dementia?

Often an individual's basic needs are overlooked, though not intentionally. It's important to remember that residents with dementia are more likely to suffer from nutritional difficulties and weight loss compared to other residents in long-term care facilities. Therefore, it's critical to make each meal time as meaningful as it can be to the patient. By establishing a common bond with a set routine, meal time will become more pleasurable and enticing.

Dementia symptoms complicate the eating process immensely. People with dementia exhibit symptoms of impaired judgment, disorientation, wandering, anxiety and memory loss. In fact, memory loss is one of the most significant dementia symptoms that affects eating. Without memory, people lose the conceptual understanding of why the body needs nourishment. An individual may not understand the purpose of eating or even recognize food for what it is.

It's important to realize that a person with dementia may be struggling with one or more of the following:

- Difficulty processing information
- Distractibility
- Poor judgment
- Decreased mobility
- Altered vision
- Altered hearing
- Poor appetite or excessive appetite
- Diminished taste and smell

Aside from the conceptual losses, dementia can result in procedural losses. Because of the confusion dementia creates, it's sometimes difficult for these individuals to even recognize that it's time to sit down for a meal. The person may even be afraid to enter the dining room. Once seated, the individual may have forgotten what the eating utensils are for and how to use them. The ability to pick up a cup or a glass may be gone.

Concepts and procedures become more unfamiliar to people with dementia as their disease progresses. This is when many patients resort to using their fingers to pick up their food. Coordinated movements—such as those required to feed yourself—may be lost as the individual's cognitive ability continues to deteriorate. A condition known as apraxia results in the patient becoming dependent on the caregiver to administer nourishment. The condition may lead to a swallowing disorder known as dysphagia, where a person may have trouble swallowing liquids, foods or saliva. In worst case scenarios, the person may be completely unable to swallow. This makes it not only difficult to eat, but also makes it difficult to take in enough calories and fluids to nourish your body.

An estimated 15 million people in the United States suffer from dysphagia, with nearly 250 million people affected around the world.(15) It's one of the leading causes of malnutrition in patients who suffer from dementia. It can be life-threatening, as people can breathe food and liquid into their lungs, aspirating the food without any visible sign of a problem. Food particles that fall into the trachea can become lodged in the lungs, causing irritation and localized swelling, which then encourages pneumonia and other pulmonary infections.

Food consistency and texture can dramatically impact dysphagia in a positive way. Individuals who may not be eating as a result of problems chewing their food may need to be shifted to a soft, pureed diet. Long-term care facility environments, however, often don't find ways to adapt their food preparation to help dysphagic individuals retain control over their eating. Instead, they simply serve bland, unidentifiable pureed foods to residents and wonder why they're not eating. Most of the time food is pureed so much that it almost becomes like soup.

Well, it doesn't have to be served that way.

Sensory-Enhanced Pureed Cuisine

With the advent of instant food thickeners, frozen pureed natural ingredients and frozen individual pureed entrees, there are ways to make this type of diet both appetizing and appealing. A phrase I coined for this is "sensory enhanced pureed cuisine." Enhancements can be used to heighten basic food color, thicken sauces and create meals with a more appealing shape and form. For example, breads can be used as a layering foundation with pureed meats, fish, chicken and vegetables. Quiches can be prepared without crusts. Cooked spinach can be replaced by a spinach soufflé roll. Even carrots can be replaced by a creamy carrot pudding along with many solid foods (*See Additional Resources,* **Websites**).

The point I'm trying to make: Meal time may be part of a routine, but the food that's central to it doesn't have to be routine. By maintaining a sense of openness, flexibility and creativity, health-care providers are finding new menu options that are compelling and satisfying. And when that happens, a more positive dining experience is created for the individual.

What needs to be present? I contend that all of the following needs to be a part of the dining experience:

- Residents need to be greeted as they enter the dining room so they feel welcome.
- Sensory stimulation: Simply put, the food needs to smell good, as well as taste good. Chafing dishes and steam tables can be used for serving food, letting the aromas fill the dining room!
- A sense of creativity: If a person has lost the ability to use utensils, then come up with creative types of finger foods to accommodate their needs.
- Tables need to be set prior to meals so the dining routine is established. If your only memory is what's in front of you, then have the dining room resemble a true dining room!
- Tabletop "conversational starters" can be as simple as 3" by 5" index cards with phrases and questions that serve as prompts for caregivers to initiate dinnertime conversation with residents. Caring Cards™ are used for this purpose.
- Have menus on the table so staff and residents know what the meal is.
- Staff should all be seated throughout the meal.
- Soft music should replace all overhead paging in the dining area.
- The color of the dishes needs to contrast with the table linens, as people with dementia have difficulty distinguishing white objects against a white background.
- Sufficient lighting so residents can see their food—and each other!

- Last, I'd like to see terry cloth protective clothing devices replaced by colorful "dining scarves"—fabric cut in the shape of a scarf and secured in the center by Velcro or snaps. A pattern is included in the back of this book (*See Additional Resources*, **Websites** and **Addendum D**). Staff must ensure that their color or fabric choices are dignified.

Dining can be an overlooked pathway when it comes to further bonding with people who have dementia. But it doesn't have to be! By making your dining room inviting, with the menu attractively displayed and careful attention paid to detail, socialization will be encouraged. Remember, this is a time that families can visit and partake in a meal with their loved ones, so their participation should also be encouraged.

In addition, staff members from all disciplines should be encouraged to get the appropriate training to enable them to assist residents during meals. This is one aspect of true culture change that will change the culture forever. By having all staff take part in assisting at meal time, everyone will have a role and the residents can benefit from the staff's conversation and companionship.

Dining can be a positive experience when common bonds are forged and positive experiences are shared. Now it's up to you to ensure that the dining experience for your residents is consistent, thoughtful and accepting.

Chapter 14
Embarking on the Final Journey

If you've followed the points I've laid out in the previous chapters—from getting to know our residents' life stories to making them feel safe, comfortable and secure in their surroundings—then you realize how critical the care you provide is to their quality of life. Just as I discussed the need for proper nutrition and nourishment in the previous chapter, I believe it's just as important—and just as vital—to provide the proper emotional nourishment throughout the final stage of a person's dementia.

It's a fact of life that Alzheimer's disease and other forms of dementia are terminal illnesses. Once a person has been diagnosed, there is no turning back. This is what makes our role as caregivers even more vital: we need to ensure that our presence and the care we provide have a positive influence on an individual until the very end.

As caregivers, our job is to provide residents with care that reduces their pain and suffering while offering them ongoing support and guidance. For a person with dementia, providing palliative care is appropriate. Palliative care places a great emphasis on reducing the severity of a disease's symptoms, regardless of one's life expectancy. Another form of palliative care is hospice care. The distinction with hospice is that it provides end-of-life care for a person who is expected to have six months or less to live.

With both palliative and hospice care, the goal is not to cure or treat the underlying disease, but rather to keep the individual as comfortable as possible by reducing pain and addressing physical, psychological, social and spiritual needs. Individuals with dementia may not outwardly exhibit a response to our care, but inside they are feeling the love we provide, which in turn enriches the quality of their lives in ways I cannot begin to describe. A person in the final stages of a terminal illness most certainly continues to benefit from experiencing life's simplest pleasures—whether it's through hearing music, smelling appealing aromas or feeling a loving caress.

Personal Example: Juliette

Earlier in my career, I had the pleasure of providing end-of-life care for a woman named Juliette who made a career for herself as a fashion designer in Paris many years ago. Juliette loved French music and all things associated with the Parisian way of life. In the final stage of her struggle with dementia, I knew we could still enrich her days by playing French music—the melodies would provide a sense of comfort and familiarity. How did I know I was making a connection? I would sit with her as she listened to the music, and she would squeeze my hand. As soon as the music stopped, her hand would go limp. It may have been the only way she could express herself, but it was a strong indicator that she was still experiencing gratification from the music she was so passionate about. By simply playing this music in her room, I was able to enrich Juliette's final days. It was gratifying to know I could still help her connect with something in life she so loved as her journey came to an end.

I believe we have untold ways within our grasp to enrich a person's life, be it physically, mentally or spiritually. A strong believer in the powers of alternative healing therapies and holistic nursing, I am a certified practitioner of Therapeutic Touch™. A contemporary interpretation of several ancient healing practices developed by Dora Kunz and Dolores Krieger, the practice is based on the assumptions that human beings are complex fields of energy—and that the ability to enhance healing in another person is a natural potential we have. Used for balancing and promoting the flow of human energy, Therapeutic Touch™ is taught in colleges worldwide and has a substantial foundation in formal and clinical research. This research has shown its usefulness in reducing pain, aiding in relaxation and easing the dying process.[16]

Personal Example: Paul

Why have I chosen to bring up Therapeutic Touch™ here? An experience I had with a gentleman named Paul and his immediate family—in this case, his wife and sister-in-law—taught me the importance of nurturing someone's spirit as well as his mind and body.

As Paul lay in his bed, we all understood the end of his life was near. Understandably, his wife had already started the grieving process, feeling that her husband had already slipped away. It was at this time that I asked if the family members would allow me to practice some Therapeutic Touch™ techniques with Paul, as well as with them. They agreed, and I'm so glad they did.

Therapeutic Touch™ has been credited with not only reducing anxiety, but also promoting a state of emotional healing. In Paul's case, his family was fraught with anxiety over what the coming days would bring. As I worked with each of them, I was able to heighten their ability to relax, accept what was taking place and make peace with the transition. Paul may not have shown it, but inside I'm sure he could experience a sense of peace. As Paul, his wife, and his sister-in-law shared this feeling together, it was surreal. Everyone felt a sense of compassion for each other, and while there was no denying that the end of Paul's life was near, there was a sense of relief in knowing that everything had been done to make the process as peaceful as possible.

As caregivers, we're used to constantly moving from room to room, always doing something to someone we're caring for. With the final stage of dementia, the most important thing we can learn to do is just "to be"—whether it's to sit next to an individual and share a good cry with them when they're feeling blue, or to take their hand in ours for a couple of precious minutes. I strongly believe that a person with dementia will feel our presence just by our being there. We all need to take a moment and remember that simply by being there, we can bring comfort to someone who's at this stage in life.

When I talk about palliative care, I cannot overemphasize the importance of the caregiver's role. On the other hand, I have to point out that the presence of distressing symptoms and difficult interventions with limited benefits is not indicative of high-quality palliative care. In fact, advanced aggressive medical treatments at the end stage of this illness—such as CPR, tube feeding, IV antibiotics and even dialysis—are of little benefit and actually may impose more suffering on the individual we should be comforting!

It's worth noting that several facilities I've worked with will not place their residents on feeding tubes to provide sustenance. This is something I firmly agree with, as studies have shown that artificial feeding does not extend the life of a person with dementia. In fact, feeding tubes not only deprive the individual of taste, but they also deprive both the person and their caregiver of personal contact, which is so essential at the final stage of life.

Granted, this is a personal choice, and one worth considering from the individual's point of view. If they could express their feelings, would they say they want this? Would they want a tube inserted into their nose, down their esophagus and into their stomach? All I'm saying is that this action merits serious reflection for people in the final stage of a terminal illness.

Through my many years of experience in the healthcare field, all too many times I've seen the ramifications of what can happen when someone doesn't make his or her wishes known regarding end of life care. This decision needs to be made at an appropriate time—and that's when a person is still able to cognitively make those decisions. If an individual's wishes are not made known prior to the onset of dementia, or at the very least during the early

A helpful resource that can guide you through the process of end of life wishes is called "Five Wishes." The document can be ordered at a minimal cost through the national non-profit organization known as Aging with Dignity. I highly recommend it. (See Additional Resources on page 115.)

stages of the diagnosis, then the person's loved one is left to make the decision. And remember, this person's caregiver is already burdened, weary and distressed by the role he or she has played.

How to Recognize When a Life Is Coming to an End

With dementia, it can be difficult to tell when death is near: people with the illness can exist in the final stage of the disease for a long period of time. However, individuals nearing the end of their lives typically show one or more of the following character-istics:

- Inability to communicate by speech
- Inability to move about without assistance
- Incontinence
- Loss of appetite
- Loss of ability to swallow
- Aspiration, pneumonia, infection or cardiac arrest (any of which can lead to a person's death)

It's important to point out that dehydration at the end state of dementia is natural—and compassionate. When a person no longer wants to eat or drink, it's a signal that the end of life is near.[17] Studies have shown that dehydration actually brings peace to the individual: as one nears death there is less fluid in the body, making it easier to breathe. As a result, the need to urinate is less frequent, and the individual will not have to be disturbed and changed as frequently. Lastly, a natural release of pain-relieving chemicals takes place in the body as it dehydrates, making the transition less painful.

The final stage of dementia is often considered a difficult time, but it doesn't have to be with the proper preparation and education. Through my work with the Connecticut Hospice, I saw first-hand how a compassionate, caring approach to dying can make the transition easier, if not peaceful. As caregivers, we need to constantly remind ourselves—and the person's family members—that the individual needs our support in life's final stages perhaps more than ever before.

Granted, it's not easy to watch someone stop eating or drinking—let alone someone we love. As caregivers, we need to work with family members to help them deal with the philosophical decisions they have to make about their loved one's life and death. By having the appropriate conversations, we can better educate and inform them about the decisions they'll have to make. Whether it's discussing issues surrounding resuscitation, tube feedings, nutrition, hydration or hospitalization, these are difficult decisions that need to be made with careful consideration by one's family members.

Given what we've just discussed, there is one question I would like you to think about: Why should a person with end-stage dementia be treated any differently than someone who has just been diagnosed with the disease? It's so important for all of us to remember that these individuals still have something to offer us—right up to the very end of their lives. That's why the roles we play in their end-of-life care are so important.

As I wrote this chapter, I was reminded of a quote from the late Scottish poet Thomas Campbell: "To live in hearts we leave behind is not to die." I believe this is the way we should all view the end of a person's life journey—by realizing that the legacy one leaves behind lives on forever.

Family members and staff alike need to take the time to celebrate a person's legacy after their passing. Remember, as professionals we have learned so many lessons from these individuals. Just think about the personal examples I've shared throughout this book: their experiences provided me with firsthand knowledge that I've woven into the fabric of my caregiving techniques.

Becoming the Path Itself

I'd like you to think once more about the quote from Buddha I used at the beginning of this book: "You cannot travel the path until you have become the path itself." The concepts I've prescribed throughout this book lay the foundation for true culture change; all we need to do is follow the path.

Think of how we've come full circle from the custodial model we had in the 1970s; no longer are there harsh consequences for individuals who don't have the ability to reason in the same way we do. Rather, by creating a culture of compassion, we can place the needs of individuals with dementia front and center and understand how we can provide caregiving that improves their quality of life and preserves their sense of dignity.

We all need to realize that a transformation of this magnitude cannot happen overnight. I'm encouraged by what I've seen through my work with facilities that commit to changing their culture. With visionary leadership and dedicated caregivers, this change will come. It requires us all to forge ahead, one day at a time, one act of compassion at a time, to build awareness and illuminate the path ahead of us.

I'm pleased that you've decided to join me on this journey.

Caring for the Caregiver

Our approach throughout the entire caregiving process—from the time of admission to the end of an individual's life—centers around the comfort, care and dignity we provide for an individual with dementia. Trust me, I'll be the first to admit that providing this level of care around the clock can take its toll on the caregiver. Our jobs require a lot from us, both physically and emotionally. That's why I'd be remiss if I didn't address how important it is for caregivers and attending staff members to receive ongoing guidance, support and positive reinforcement so they feel their work is valued.

As caregivers, we need to feel we are essential if this new culture is to thrive; we need to know that our opinions are respected, that our work with residents is appreciated and that our needs are understood. I know that this disease is difficult; patience, kindness and empathy are key. But I also know there are times when we have to take a "time out" to remind ourselves why we're here and to get the support we need.

We spend so much of our time at work that it's natural for us to form relationships with our colleagues. That's why it's important for us to do periodic check-ins with each other. We need to know that we can talk to each other and recognize when stress is taking its toll; when we see one of our colleagues starting to lose tolerance, for example, we need to take them off to the side and ask what we can do to help. If we want to create a caring culture, we have to start with ourselves and our colleagues. After all, if we're not there for each other, then how can we be there for the people under our care?

Remember, as a caregiver, self care isn't a luxury—it is a necessity!

Taking the Staff Lounge One Step Further

A long-term care facility's top priority should be to create an environment where its staff can receive the nurturing it needs in order to provide quality care for its residents. In the old days, a facility would designate an area for its staff lounge and say they had done what they needed to do in providing a break area for staff members. Well, under this new culture, it takes a lot more than a staff lounge to provide the physical and emotional nourishment a well-trained caregiving staff needs.

For example, we need to designate a quiet area where caregivers can relax, unwind and decompress. If you manage such a facility, look at your current staff lounge and think about how you can make it more accommodating. Is there an area where a caregiver can go to meditate for a few minutes? Are there breathing exercises you can provide them with? Is there an area where they can listen to music for a few minutes to calm down and renew themselves? Are there massaging chairs that can help alleviate their stress and relax them? Simply put, facilities need to understand how to best care for the caregivers on their staff if they want to provide quality care for their residents.

It's important to emphasize that the changes I prescribe don't require a significant investment. Here are some simple suggestions that can help a facility provide better care for its staff:

- *Listen to your staff's needs.* You need to do periodic "check-ins" with your staff and offer channels through which they can make their concerns known. By being sensitive to their needs, you'll help them not only alleviate their problems, but also offer more compassionate care for your residents.

- *Offer team support groups.* Preventing staff burnout should be your No. 1 priority aside from providing quality care for your residents. By scheduling regular support group meetings, you can create a culture where your caregivers feel their needs are being met. For example, you could bring in guest speakers specializing in stress reduction methods, Therapeutic Touch™ or breathing techniques, to name a few.

- *Schedule ongoing education/training/workshops.* Caregivers often need to develop skills that simply are not being taught. Look for ways to get creative with your schedules and make it a priority to include time for regular training. Keep in mind that training doesn't need to be led by an outside facilitator; some of the role playing exercises I've mentioned in this book can accomplished in an hour or less. Just allowing staff to put themselves in a resident's shoes for an afternoon can be one of the best learning experiences!

- *Prominently display resources available to staff.* Caregivers should not have to look very hard to find information that can help them do their jobs better. By making such resources as books, websites and audio training classes available to your staff, you'll be giving them sources of guidance they otherwise may not be able to access.

Remember, the national Alzheimer's Association website has numerous free tools and services available, including online courses, a virtual library, caregiving tips and strategies, a stress checklist, training opportunities, message boards and personal stories. Just think about the resources we have at our disposal today compared to when Alzheimer's disease was discovered more than 100 years ago. With many resources just the click of a mouse away, we can no longer say it's too expensive or time-consuming to provide this information for our staff.

Epilogue
Four Kinds of People in This World

Former First Lady Rosalynn Carter summed it best when she said: "There are only four kinds of people in the world—those who have been caregivers, those who are currently caregivers, those who will be caregivers and those who will need caregivers."

We only get to travel this path once, and as Mrs. Carter said, it's likely that in our lifetime we will find ourselves in need of the care that we are striving now to provide. As we've discussed in this book, we can only begin to know what it's like for a person with dementia by taking the time to walk in their shoes.

From now on, when we embark on our walk together, it's our responsibility to make sure the shoes are a perfect fit.

Sources

(1)   2011 Alzheimer's Disease Facts and Figures, Alzheimer's Association.

(2)   Nation's First Baby Boomer Files for Social Security Retirement Benefits—
        Online, Social Security Administration Press Release, October 15, 2007.

(3),(10) Assisted Living State Regulatory Review 2010, National Center for
        Assisted Living. Retrieved March 2010, from
        http://tinyurl.com/2dt6n7o.

(4)   Notes Towards a Definition of Culture, T.S. Eliot, 1948.

(5)   Alzheimer's Association of Connecticut Chapter.

(6)   Alzheimer's and Dementia: Brain Structure, American Academy of
        Neurology, April 17, 2007.

(7)   Communication Difficulties: Assessment and Interventions in
        Hospitalized Older Adults with Dementia, Try This, Issue #D7,
        Revised 2007, published by The John A. Hartford Institute for Geriatric
        Nursing and the Alzheimer's Association.

(8)   Experiencing Life, Briefly, Inside a Nursing Home, The New York Times,
        April 23, 2009.

(9)   Turnaround or Shutdown: A Small Town Facility Worth Saving, used with
        permission from Vigilan Inc. Retrieved from
        http://www.vigilan.com/pdfs/case_studies/Turnaround3.pdf.

(11)   A Practical Program for Preventing Delirium in Hospitalized Elderly
        Patients, Take-home Points from Lectures by Cleveland Clinic and Visiting
        Faculty, Cleveland Clinic Journal of Medicine, Vol. 71, No. 11, November
        2005. Retrieved from http://tinyurl.com/6yznfls.

(12)   Consolidating Medication Passes, American Journal of Nursing, Volume
        105(12), December 2005.

(13)   Paro Theraupetic Robot. http://www.parorobots.com.

(14)   Emotions Outlast the Memories that Drive Them, National Public Radio.
        April 13, 2010.

(15)   Life with Dysphagia, eSwallow USA, LLC. http://www.eswallow.net.

(16)   Therapeutic Touch Defined, Pumpkin Hollow Association. Retrieved
        December 2004, from http://www.therapeutictouch.org.

(17)   Patient Refusal of Nutrition and Hydration: Walking the Ever-Finer Line,
        American Journal Hospice & Palliative Care. March/April 1995.

Additional Resources
Articles

An Overview of Therapeutic Touch and Its Application to Patients with Alzheimer's Disease, *American Journal of Alzheimer's Disease*, Vol. 13, No. 4, July/August 1998

Culinary Strategies Help Residents with Dysphagia Regain Dignity, *Provider Magazine*, October 199s

Factors Contributing to Minimizing Weight Loss in Patients with Dementia, *The American Journal of Alzheimer's Disease*, Vol. 10, No. 4, July/August 1995

Using Family Style Meals to Increase Participation and Communication in Persons with Dementia, *Journal of Gerontological Nursing*, November 2002

Books

Core Curriculum for Professional Education in Pain, Third Edition, ISAP Press 2011

Hard Choices for Loving People, Hank Dunn, A&A Publishers Inc. 2001

Websites

Alzheimer's Association	www.alz.org
Aging with Dignity	www.agingwithdignity.org
Hartford Institute for Geriatric Nursing	www.consultgerirn.org
Lippincott's Nursing Center	www.nursingcenter.com
The C.A.R.E. Channel	www.healinghealth.com
Enhanced Vision	www.enhancedvision.com
Reflection Connection	www.reflectionconnection.net
The Validation Training Institute, Inc.	www.vfvalidation.org
Sound Oasis® sleep therapy pillow	www.sound-oasis.com
Brookstone, functional products	www.brookstone.com
Vision Simulations	www.visionsimulations.com
NoiseMeters Inc.	www.noisemeters.com
Super Brush	www.superbrush.com
Therapeutic Touch™	www.therapeutictouch.org
Professional Fit Clothing	www.professionalfit.com
Caring Cards™	www.dramycaregiving.com/store
Fractiles®	www.fractiles.com
Sensory-Enhanced Cuisine, recipes	www.randy-griffin.com

(DTNA)
Dementia Training Needs Analysis

The Dementia Training Needs Analysis is designed to help you identify the programmatic and environmental elements needed to successfully implement the "Relationship-Based Dementia Care Model," also referred to as the "New Culture in Dementia Care and Culture Change." This model focuses on the restoration of wholeness and emphasizes the importance of the body/mind/spirit integration, regardless of whether the pathology is eliminated. The relationship-based model assumes that in any relationship, both parties have something of value to give and receive. From this perspective, caregivers are encouraged to take an empathy-based approach where they see the person with dementia as a human being, similar to themselves.

Research has shown that long-term facilities, based on the medical model, often neglect or minimize the core social and emotional needs of people that are central to the Relationship-Based Dementia Care Model.

The Dementia Training Needs Analysis (DTNA) tool has been developed to:
1. Focus on the strengths of the organization
2. Identify areas for potential growth
3. Identify education and training needs
4. Provide the basis for the development of a tailored Dementia Training Program

The DTNA provides for a self-analysis in three domains:
E= Environment
S= Social and Emotional Connection
P= Physical Comfort

Instructions

The DTNA is an observational tool. To achieve maximum validity, the person(s) completing the tool should collect multiple observations (e.g., multiple shifts, locations, observe different staff at different times of the day). Observations should be collected until you are comfortable that you have a good representation of the facility.

For each item on the scale check whether the item is:

☐ Frequently Observed
☐ Periodically Observed
☐ Not Observed

You're encouraged to make notes in the comments area where appropriate.

Facility Name: _____

Dates: _____
(Time period of assessment)

Name of Team reviewer: _____

Team members being assessed: _____
(Nursing, Recreation, Food and Nu-
trition, Social Service, Housekeeping,
Maintenance, Laundry, other):

Shifts: _____

Focus Area: *Environment*

Intention—The environment supports the person with dementia. From the time you enter the designated space you should get the distinct feeling that there is something special about the unit that distinguishes it from other units in the facility.

Before answering the specific questions on the next pages, jot down your first impressions of the environment; if you were walking into this area for the first time, what would stand out for you

_____

_____

_____

_____

_____

Environmental Factor	Practice is consistently observed	Practice is periodically observed	Practice is not observed	Comments/Observations
The Unit is quiet. Loud, distracting noises are minimized.				
Staff minimizes noise/communications that are not intended to be direct communications with the residents ☐ Overhead paging ☐ Walkie-talkies ☐ Cell phones for personal conversations				
Staff limits the number of residents with chair alarms; when alarms do go off they respond as quickly as possible.				
Staff speaks quietly to both residents and each other.				
Televisions that are turned on are actually being watched, and are set to appropriate channels.				
Music playing in common areas is soft and used as background music.				
Carts on the unit, such as medication carts, linen carts and food carts, are well maintained and do not make loud or annoying noises.				
Cleaning is scheduled to minimize disruption to unit activities; vacuums and other cleaning equipment noises are low.				
Staff minimizes other loud noises such as medication crushing and banging of doors.				
Places for quiet and solitude are available on the unit for residents.				

The Unit is visually pleasing, welcoming and appropriate for the residents (May want to do separate ratings for different areas such as activity room, dining area, hallways).

Environmental Factor	Practice is consistently observed	Practice is periodically observed	Practice is not observed	Comments/Observations
Lighting is adequate for low vision.				
The space includes some form of visual welcoming, such as a sign or a basket of flowers, which differentiates it from other spaces in the building.				
The unit has adequate indirect lighting (e.g., table or floor lamps, recessed lights above bedroom doorways, windows, skylights).				
Lighting is used to help individuals with day and night cues.				
Dimmers are used to provide lighting for quiet time and relaxation for naps or sleep.				
Contrasting color is used in the hallways.				
Contrasting color is used on walls, toilets, sinks, baths or showers.				
Railings are in a contrasting color from the wall.				
Glare is minimized (e.g., floors are not shined to the point where they produce glare).				
Shower rooms are inviting, pleasant and home-like.				

119

Environmental Factor	Practice is consistently observed	Practice is periodically observed	Practice is not observed	Comments/Observations
Colors in the bathroom and/or shower rooms are calming and inviting.				
Carpets are simple not overly busy and patterned.				
Photos, signage and other wall hangings are positioned for those who are ambulatory as well as in wheelchairs.				
Signage is visible for people to see pictures and clues (e.g., bold letters, bright contrast, three-dimensional).				
Signage is used to identify different rooms.				
Live plants and flowers are visible on the unit.				
The resident's room is personalized through furniture, pictures and objects. The room itself tells a story about who the person is.				
The Unit is structured to foster interaction with the residents.				
The nursing station is not the center of activity and, when possible, has been removed.				
Seating areas are provided on the unit for conversation or rest areas.				
The furniture placement is done with purpose. Furniture is arranged to take advantage of window views.				

120

Environmental Factor	Practice is consistently observed	Practice is periodically observed	Practice is not observed	Comments/Observations
The facility has a space (e.g., café, lounge, ice cream parlor) for families, visitors and residents to mingle and socialize outside the unit or neighborhood.				
The unit includes discovery stations for staff, visitors and family to interact with the resident.				
Raised gardens are available.				
The facility has an outdoor garden; walking and wheeling paths are accessible.				
Dining				
The dining room is decorated as a dining room.				
If the dining room is used as a multipurpose room, the tables are pre-set before meals.				
Meals are served on time so that residents are not left waiting for long periods of time.				
Tables include tablecloths and/or placemats and a centerpiece.				
Plates are a different color from the table or mats.				
Background music is playing during the meal.				
Food is served either buffet style, family style or through table service (not with trays being placed on the tables).				

Environmental Factor	Practice is consistently observed	Practice is periodically observed	Practice is not observed	Comments/Observations
Dining hours last at least 2 hrs to encourage socialization.				
Caregivers are seated during the meal time hour.				
Dishes are scraped in the kitchen, not in the dining room.				
Medications are not administrated during the meal hour.				
Nursing, recreation and other trained staff are available during meals. Staff breaks and meals are not scheduled during resident meal times.				
Staff converse with residents rather than exclusively with each other during meals.				
Pureed foods are served in an attractive manner.				
Tables are clean and clutter free.				
Dignified protective cloths are used during the meal hour.				
Caregivers frequently wipe resident's mouth w/napkins.				
Staff partakes in dining with the residents to make it a social event.				

Environmental Factor	Practice is consistently observed	Practice is periodically observed	Practice is not observed	Comments/Observations
Finger foods are available as needed; bread is always available to make finger food sandwiches.				
Residents are not placed at a table according to a prescribed food consistency.				
Pantries with refrigerators are accessible to staff for the residents and their families.				

Focus Area: *Social and Emotional Connection*

Intention—Caregivers communicate effectively with residents. Meaningful social engagement can be highly pleasurable for residents and can open up a whole new dimension to their daily lives. Caregivers need to understand the impact of verbal and non-verbal language and should be familiar with a resident's life history.

Before answering the specific questions below, jot down your first impressions of how you see staff interacting with residents.

_____

_____

_____

_____

_____

Social and Emotional Connection Factor	Practice is consistently observed	Practice is periodically observed	Practice is not observed	Comments/Observations
Active engagement is seen on the unit.				
Staff spend time listening and conversing with residents.				
When addressing the resident, the caregiver uses the resident's first and/or last name.				
The caregiver maintains eye contact while conversing with the resident.				
The caregiver knows many details about the personal history of the resident.				
The caregiver carries on conversations with residents while performing activities of daily living. This conversation speaks to the person, what they enjoy, and uses pieces from their past.				
Staff have sufficient access to personal information about residents (e.g., past and present hobbies, things they enjoy) to support meaningful individualized engagements.				
Assignment sheets include important facts from the personal history of the resident.				

Social and Emotional Connection Factor	Practice is consistently observed	Practice is periodically observed	Practice is not observed	Comments/Observations
Assignment sheets include critical information to inform staff as to the communication needs of residents including: • Resident can read • Resident can understand pictures • Resident understands yes and no • Resident uses automatic language (yes and no) without understanding meaning • Resident has past visual age-related problems • Resident needs glasses for distance or reading • Resident uses hearing aids				
Music assessments are completed on each resident upon admission.				
Staff uses songs as an intervention while caring for residents and knows residents' favorite songs.				
Staff uses positive language with the resident.				
Staff do not use negative labels such as "the feeder," "the total," "the hitter," "the screamer," "the wanderer," etc.				
Staff is aware of and, where possible, communicates with residents in their primary language.				
To the extent possible residents exercise control over their own schedules (e.g, being bathed as often as they like).				

126

Social and Emotional Connection Factor	Practice is consistently observed	Practice is periodically observed	Practice is not observed	Comments/Observations
Past histories involving all personal care is discussed. Details such as bathing time and preferences, bedtime and awake-time hours are known.				
Life histories are shared with other team members.				
Resident's birthdays are celebrated on the day of, in addition to any monthly celebrations.				
Programming/Activities				
Activities and programs are based on life histories.				
Programs are designed with a specific goal for each resident.				
Programs are developed to meet the needs of residents with special adaptations.				
The unit's interdisciplinary team (including Nursing, Recreation, Housekeeping, Laundry, Dietary, Social Service, PT and OT) meets on a regular basis.				
All disciplines take responsibility for social, emotional and spiritual activities. Staff from diverse disciplines, including nursing and recreation, conducts programs.				
Residents connect with nature at least 3 times a week.				

127

Social and Emotional Connection Factor	Practice is consistently observed	Practice is periodically observed	Practice is not observed	Comments/Observations
Family involvement is encouraged. Family programming is offered to families at different hours and on weekends.				
Activities involving families, residents and staff are core programs.				
Programming is offered 7 days per week.				
Programming begins by 10 am and continues until 8 pm.				
Physical exercise is encouraged through dance, chair yoga, stretching, passive and active.				
Programming includes: • Community involvement • Day trips • Intergenerational programming • Activities that encourage creative self-expression, involving the senses, emotions and imagination • Activities involving animals such as dogs or cats • Large and small groups, as well as one-on-one activities				
A facility-wide volunteer program supports the Dementia Care Unit and is seen as part of the existing culture.				
Staff from other departments volunteer on the Dementia Care Unit by serving as new friend, angel, buddy, adopted grandparent, etc.				

128

Focus Area: *Physical Comfort*

Intention—Caregivers effectively provide for residents' physical comfort.
Physical comfort includes seeing to the physical needs in an attentive and respectful manner. It also includes addressing pain and providing compassionate palliative care.

Before answering the specific questions below, jot down your first impressions of how you see staff interacting with residents.

_____

_____

_____

_____

_____

Physical Comfort Factor	Practice is consistently observed	Practice is periodically observed	Practice is not observed	Comments/Observations
Caregivers listen and observe for any signs of distress.				
Caregivers observe residents during all ADL's for pain or discomfort.				
The unit uses a dementia-screening tool for pain.				
The unit offers non-pharmacological modalities for pain, such as Therapeutic Touch™, Reiki, massage and reflexology.				
Caregivers demonstrate an understanding of both emotional and physical pain.				
Pain indicators are clearly defined.				
Residents are not medicated for pain to the point where it impairs other functioning (e.g., communication).				
Palliative Care				
Staff understands the nature and approach of palliative care.				
Staff continues to attend to emotional and physical comfort needs when a resident is actively dying.				
Staff provides help with grief and loss after a person has died.				
Staff has a ritual that honors the person who has passed away upon their death.				

130

Physical Comfort Factor	Practice is consistently observed	Practice is periodically observed	Practice is not observed	Comments/Observations
The facility arranges for a staff member to be with the person unless family or friends are available or the resident has made it known that they would rather be alone.				
Families of dying residents have an adequately equipped place to stay in the facility (e.g, bed to sleep in, linens, a place to dress and shower).				
The Dietary Team offers an adequately stocked and maintained comfort cart filled with food, beverages, etc. to meet the needs of the families.				

Training Factor	Practice is consistently observed	Practice is periodically observed	Practice is not observed	Comments/Observations
Training/Supervision				
The facility mandates at least 12 hours of annual Dementia Care Education for anyone working on the unit.				
The facility mandates at least 12 hours of annual Dementia Care Education for Dining Room staff.				
The facility offers specialized training in hand and foot massage, Therapeutic Touch, Aromatherapy, Reiki and other non-pharmacological practices.				
The facility requires training in Palliative Care.				
The facility offers/requires a specialized training class for staff from outside agencies (e.g., per diems).				
Members of the Dementia Team are cross-trained to help in dining and programming.				
Staff is assigned permanent shifts.				
Pain education is part of the Dementia Care Training Program.				

132

Addendum A
Conversational Starters

When speaking to people with Dementia, recall can be most challenging and difficult. With these conversational starters, we are not trying to test their memories, but instead we are looking for ways to engage them in meaningful conversation. Look at the examples of how questions can be re-designed to promote conversation with easy yes and no responses.

- What did you have for lunch today? Did you enjoy your meal?
- What did you do all day? The day is really going by fast!
- What would you like to do now? Would you like to take a walk?
- Is that a new sweater? What a beautiful sweater! I don't remember it, it must be new. Beautiful color!
- Do you know who I am? I am [____] I am glad to see you !
- Do you want to watch any special program on TV? Let's see if there is anything on TV that you may like to watch.
- Did you get your hair done today? Your hair looks beautiful!
- You just told me that! That sounds interesting! I would like to hear more about that!
- What kind of work did you do? You must have been very good at your job.

Words to use to show that you are listening:
- I see
- How interesting
- Is that so?
- Did it?
- How nice
- Sounds like a great idea
- I see what you mean
- I heard of that
- Really
- Thanks for sharing that

Addendum B
Getting to Know You

1. What is your full name? Do you have a nickname?
2. Where were you born?
3. What is your favorite season of the year? What makes it your favorite?
4. What month were you born? What was the best birthday celebration you can recall? What made it so special?
5. Tell me about a hobby you really enjoy doing.
6. Have you ever shared this hobby with another person?
7. If you were asked to teach other friends something that you are passionate about, what would it be?
8. What kind of music do you like? Do you have a favorite song? Can you name a childhood song that you recall? What favorite instrument do you play? Did you ever take music lessons? Tell me more about this.
9. Help me finish this sentence: Joy and happiness for me have come from _____.
10. Do you like to garden? What type of flowers do you like? What color flowers?
11. Do you like to take walks? Tell me about a place you love taking walks.
12. If you had a day to spend any way you wanted, and money was not a factor, what would you do? If you could take one person with you, who would you take and why?
13. Tell me about a project you did with your own two hands.
14. Do you like sports? Was there a favorite sport you did as a child? Teen? Adult?
15. What is your favorite holiday tradition?
16. What kind of home do you live in? What is your favorite room in the house and why?
17. What type of pets did you have as a child? Adult?
18. What irritates you? What do you do to manage distress?
19. Who in your early adult life inspired you?

20. What critical life event helped to shape you?
21. Tell me a color that makes you feel great when you wear it or see it?
22. What do you do to renew your energy?
23. Tell me about a time where incredible faith was required of you?
24. Tell me two accomplishments in your life that you are most proud of?
25. What provides you with a feeling of comfort? For example, a piece of clothing, a scent of perfume, a favorite song, a comfort food.
26. What has been your favorite vacation?
27. What is your best friend's name? What are some of the qualities that best describe your friend?
28. When you are troubled, sad and your energy is low, what do you do to get yourself feeling better?
29. What is it that you most want to be appreciated for?

Addendum C
Pain Assessment IN Advanced Dementia
PAINAD

	0	1	2	Score
Breathing Independent of vocalization	Normal	Occasional labored breathing. Short period of hyperventilation	Noisy labored breathing. Long period of hyperventilation. Cheyne-strokes respirations	
Negative Vocalization	None	Occasional moan or groan. Low level of speech with a negative or disapproving quality	Repeated troubled calling out. Loud moaning or groaning. Crying	
Facial expression	Smiling, or inexpressive	Sad. Frightened. Frown	Facial grimacing	
Body Language	Relaxed	Tense. Distressed pacing. Fidgeting	Rigid. Fists clenched, Knees pulled up. Pulling or pushing away. Striking out.	
Consolability	No need to console	Distracted or reassured by voice or touch	Unable to console, distract or reassure.	
				Total

The PAINAD was developed and tested by clinicians and researchers at the New England Geriatric Research Education and Clinical Center, a Department of Veterans Affairs center of excellence with divisions at EN Rogers Memorial Veterans Hospital, Bedford, MA, and VA Boston Health System. We are committed to maintaining the validity and reliability of the PAINAD as a clinical and research tool.

Additional suggested instrument for assessment: NOPPAIN
Non-Communicative Patient's Pain Assessment Instrument.
http://prc.coh.org/PainNOA/NOPPAIN_Tool.pdf

Addendum D
Dining Scarf

Instructions and tips for creating Dining Scarves
Used with Permission by Jan Baker, developer of the Jaclean Dining Scarf

Cut the pattern with the neck end on the fold of pattern paper, or cut two and tape them together. I suggest using thin poster board cardboard for the pattern. You may want to make multiple patterns for cutting large numbers at one time.

Chose fabric that is 100% polyester in bright colors and patterns. This fabric usually comes in 58"–60" width. It should be wrinkle free and scarf weight but have enough stability to cover clothing adequately when lying flat. Too heavy fabrics and cottons will give a result that looks bib like and are considered unsuitable. Too flimsy will not lie flat for dining. Patterns and florals are especially nice.

The final pattern is one side of the full scarf. Cut two per scarf. I suggest buying fabrics by the bolt, possibly from areas like NYC which often sells bolts or large bolt ends for about $2 per yard. The bolts can be rolled out on a long wide table and then go back and forth, layering the fabric so that many can be cut at one time. (Or on a narrower table, fold the fabric exactly in half and then layer.) Electric scissors or very sharp fabric scissors are recommended. Place multiple patterns on the fabric and use weights to hold them in place. Place patterns as close as possible to get maximum numbers of scarves on the fabric.

After cutting, place two halves right sides together and stitch around each one leaving a four inch space open for turning, (usually on one of the neck sides) clip corners, trim seam on curves. Top stitch this neck area. Some people top stitch the entire scarf but this is optional and might lessen the scarf-like appearance on some fabrics.

The dimensions of the dining scarf fit most people but some very large obese people require a larger and longer scarf.

The dining scarves are stain resistant. Before laundering some stains, especially on solid fabrics, might require Spray and Wash or some product which releases the food or oil spills.

Dining scarves are not waterproof. If a more waterproof dining scarf is desired, choose very light waterproof nylon material that is used for windbreakers and lightweight raingear as a lining fabric for the scarf excluding the neck area. It may be placed in the lower area of each end of the scarf and stitched in on the wrong side of the fabric before turning.

Adding Grace and Beauty to Mealtime

This easy sewing pattern creates a dignified way to help people stay clean at meal times and during the day. Get creative and have fun with selecting different fabric colors and prints and changing the pattern dimensions to make it wider, longer or thinner. We have found that 100% Polyester fabric seems to work the best. Wrapping paper or paper from office type flip charts works well to cut the pattern from.

10 Easy Steps to Sewing a Dining Scarf

1. Fold your fabric in half.
2. Place pattern on the fold of the fabric. Cut 2 patterns for 1 scarf. This will make the 2 panels for the front and back of the scarf.
3. Turn the fabric inside out (colorful side will be on the inside and the back of the fabric will be facing outside).
4. When opening the fabric, you will have a long scarf.
5. Before sewing, decide which will be the top and bottom of the scarf. (Both will look the same).
6. With both pattern pieces together, sew along the outer edge, making a ¼" seam and leave a 4" opening on the bottom of the scarf. (This is to allow turning the scarf right side out).
7. Clip curve in corners to release tension on the fabric.
8. Iron the scarf.
9. Turn the scarf right side out.
10. Tuck in 1/4 " of the bottom opening and sew it, continuing to sew around the entire scarf to hold the front and back fabric together securely to avoid bunching.

Dining Scarf Pattern

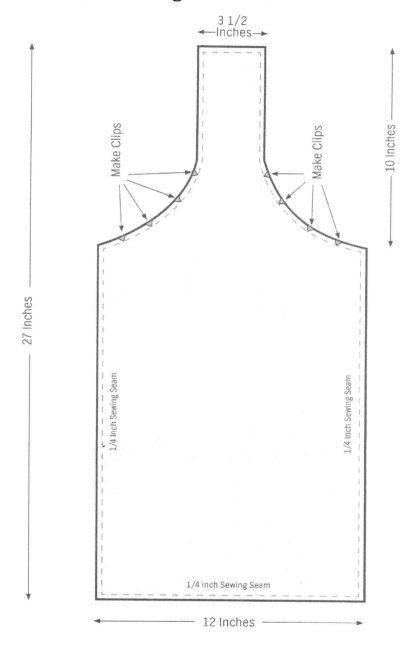

Used with permission by Jan Baker, developer of the Jaclean Dining Scarf

About the Author

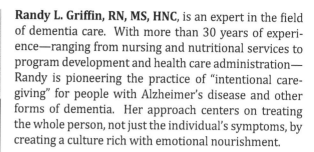

Randy L. Griffin, RN, MS, HNC, is an expert in the field of dementia care. With more than 30 years of experience—ranging from nursing and nutritional services to program development and health care administration—Randy is pioneering the practice of "intentional caregiving" for people with Alzheimer's disease and other forms of dementia. Her approach centers on treating the whole person, not just the individual's symptoms, by creating a culture rich with emotional nourishment.

Randy's programs and models have set new standards in caring for patients with Alzheimer's disease and related dementias while educating their families and caregivers. Randy recently developed "The Trusting Touch," a Webinar that teaches the importance of intentional actions and verbal communications during such activities as bathing, dressing and dental care. Randy also is the author of "S.A.F.E. Response Techniques in Crisis Situations," a four-step process to show staff how to safely handle agitation and address aggressive behaviors when caring for people with dementia. In addition, Randy has developed innovative dining programs for people with Alzheimer's disease and other forms of dementia.

Earlier in her career, Randy was the Director of Nutritional Services for the Connecticut Hospice, the first free-standing hospice in the U.S. While working for the hospice, she developed one of the first sensory-enhanced puréed cuisine culinary programs for terminally ill individuals. She also authored the first published cookbook on the formation of sensory-enhanced purées. Later, Randy was the Associate Director of the Alzheimer's Resource Center and also served as its Director of Education, Training and Research. Her background in nursing and culinary training as a chef in Paris provided the impetus for her innovative approaches to nursing care, dining creations and culture change for long-term care facilities. "Dining with Grace" is one of the programs she created specifically to enhance the dining experience for people with Alzheimer's disease and other forms of dementia.

Randy is a Certified Holistic Nurse, Reflexologist and Therapeutic Touch™ practitioner and instructor. Randy's latest DVD "An Introduction to Therapeutic Touch" will be released January 2012.

Recognized as an expert in the fields of dementia and hospice care, Randy lectures and leads workshops nationwide while providing consulting services to health care facilities. For more information about Randy, please visit: www.randy-griffin.com

36590922R00088

Made in the USA
Lexington, KY
26 October 2014